A DIETITIAN'S CANCER STORY

Information and Inspiration for Recovery and Healing from a 3-Time Cancer Survivor

Diana Dyer, MS, RD
Swan Press
Ann Arbor, MI

The information presented in this book describes the author's personal recovery path after her second breast cancer diagnosis. It is not intended to be individualized medical or nutritional advice. Please discuss and advocate for your own needs and choices related to nutrition, cancer treatment, recovery, prevention, and optimal wellness with your team of health care professionals, which should include a Registered Dietitian (RD).

ISBN 978-0-9667238-3-0
Library of Congress Catalog Card Number 00-190231

First printing, June 1997.
Second printing, July 1997.
Third printing, September 1997.
Fourth printing, April 1998.
Fifth printing, February 1999.
Sixth printing, August 2000.
Seventh printing, January 2001.
Eighth printing, March 2002.
Ninth printing, December 2003.
Tenth printing, April 2005.
Eleventh printing, October 2007.
Twelfth printing, March 2010

Logo design by Janus Productions
Layout by Graham W. Burns
Cover Design by Dorothea Goodwin

To my family
whose continuous love is the reason I did not give up
after my third cancer diagnosis

☙ TABLE OF CONTENTS

- Sample Menus
- Travel Tips—Ideas for Eating on the Road or Bringing Your Own Food
- Conclusion

- Nature
- Support Groups
- Cancer Survivors' Network
- Exercise, including T'ai Chi and Qi Gong
- Homeopathy
- Meditation
- Guided Imagery
- Hypnotherapy
- Feng Shui
- Shiatsu
- Prayer
- Reading
- Gardening

- My Website—www.CancerRD.com
- Frequently Asked Questions
  - FAQ #1   I have just been diagnosed with cancer. What steps do you suggest I take?
  - FAQ #2   Do you ever "cheat" on your diet?
  - FAQ #3   What do you eat for snacks?
  - FAQ #4   Does sugar "feed" tumors?
  - FAQ #5   Is your shake recipe really just one serving? Can I save it for later?
  - FAQ #6   My blender won't blend the carrots. Do you have suggestions?
  - FAQ #7   Can herbs interact with any of the chemotherapy drugs?
  - FAQ #8   Which herbs might cause problems with blood clotting?

ABOUT THE COVER

The new cover design for the 2002 edition of my book represents a compilation of several meaningful aspects of my life. While I have always felt connected to small lakes, ponds, and swans, I had two healing experiences that brought these loves together after my cancer diagnosis in 1995. While meditating one morning, I had an unanticipated "vision" that large flocks of swans were flying into my body on my breath to help me fight this cancer. On another occasion, five Trumpeter swans unexpectedly visited the small pond in my neighborhood. After years of going elsewhere to look for swans, on those two special days they came to me.

The colors used in the background on the book cover are similar to those I have seen during sunrises, when meditating at the beginning of a day. I am grateful for the moment of seeing the sunrise, knowing that God has given me the gift of being alive another day, a truly delicious moment.

Meditating on a bridge represents where I have found myself professionally; on a bridge between the two worlds of conventional and alternative health care. It is my hope that the future will have just one health care system, blending the best of both approaches to provide the most effective and comprehensive patient care.

As I pondered several possible cover designs and designers for the new 2002 edition of my book, my heart led me to Dorothea Goodwin, a local artist who created the design for the headstone on my father's grave. Dorothea sensitively interwove many meaningful personal aspects of my father's life into that etching, and I intuitively knew she would do the same for my book cover, too.

My first meditation instructor, Janus Winger, developed my logo in 1997. Incorporating my love of swans, the upward arrow between the two swans represents the opportunity that a cancer diagnosis presents to have a new beginning each day while traveling both forward and upward on life's journey. The logo is as meaningful to me today as it was then.

FOREWORD

As a three-time cancer survivor as well as a health care professional, Diana Dyer offers unique perspectives on various complementary approaches to improve the quality of life in cancer patients. These approaches include lifestyle changes such as diet, exercise, meditation, as well as other techniques that should be viewed not as alternatives to conventional medicine, but rather as complementary. Furthermore, these strategies may be of value not only during the active treatment of cancer, but also during the period of recovery. By becoming active participants in these lifestyle changes, as Diana has done, cancer survivors can better regain control of their lives and improve its quality. The information in this booklet should be valuable to cancer survivors and their families.

Max Wicha, MD, Director
The University of Michigan Comprehensive Cancer Center
Ann Arbor, Michigan

COMMENTS

A sampling of comments I have received from individuals after attending my public speaking presentations, watching my TV appearances, or reading my book.

"Because of my family history of breast cancer, I don't know what the future will bring, and frankly, I am sometimes frightened. But what has amazed me is the large number of women I have met who have experienced this illness and how they are LIVING! I really appreciated the opportunity to hear you speak. Thank you for sharing your journey."

"Our group has never given anyone else a standing ovation!"

"I was very touched and motivated by your story."

"One can't help being impressed with your interesting and informative book which catches the poignancy of your cancer experiences and life changes."

"Your life story is an inspiration to us all. You truly spoke to my heart."

"Your talk was one of the very best programs we have ever had presented."

"Saw you on TV. You were wonderful and inspiring. Thank you!"

"Thank you for your valuable information. I truly believe you are right."

"Thank you for the efforts you are making to help us. Keep up the good work."

"You are giving cancer survivors real hope. Thank you for reaching out."

"I would just like to say how interesting I found your television appearance today. It was refreshing to watch someone so down to earth and pleasant, rather than a "know-it-all" or "super-person" like so many. No doubt, your practicality has helped you to get through your ordeals."

"All 70,000 members of the American Dietetic Association should own this book."

Preface to the 1998 Printing

So much has happened in my life during the past year since the *Detroit Free Press* published an article about my cancer recovery. I was invited to be on national TV, interviewed by many newspapers, the keynote speaker for a "Race for the Cure," spoke to numerous cancer survivor groups, professional conferences for various health care professionals, and Medical Grand Rounds at major medical centers, along with being honored by my state professional organization (Michigan Dietetic Association) with its Individual Public Relations Award. In addition, I've had the opportunity to meet Jane Brody, author and health writer for *The New York Times*, and, I have received a hand-written note from Dr. Bernie Siegel, author of *Love, Medicine, and Miracles*. Amazement is an understatement!

However, writing and revising this book, along with mailing it out to each of you who have ordered it, have given me the greatest sense of both pleasure and contentment. I thank all of my readers, whom I think of as new friends, for the constant support and encouragement that so many of you have sent to me via telephone calls, letters, E-mail, and prayers. I also admire all of you and encourage you to start writing and speaking of your own inspirational stories that you have so openly told me.

I would like to share the quote that I often use to end my speaking presentations. It so clearly expresses my sense of amazement and wonder at what has happened to me after my latest cancer diagnosis:

> *"Every journey has a secret destination of which the traveler is unaware."*—Martin Buber

My hope for you is that your own cancer journey will also lead you to unexpected, but surprisingly wonderful, people, places, and opportunities.

With warmest regards,
Diana Dyer

April 1998

Preface to the 1999 Printing

My vision for the distribution of *A Dietitian's Cancer Story* has been to have it available in cancer centers across the country to be given to cancer patients. I wrote this book to be just what I wish my own cancer center would have given me when I started asking the question, "What else can I be doing to help with my recovery?" It is a concise guide to strategies that may help enhance the benefit of conventional cancer therapies. It also helps a newly diagnosed patient learn various techniques for becoming an equal partner in his or her cancer care and an informed consumer of complementary medicine.

Bulk pricing is available for quantity orders of my book. Several cancer centers have done this already, and one cancer center bought enough for all of their patients to have an individual copy. Memorial gift funds have been used to purchase these books, which has been very meaningful to me.

A significant percentage of the proceeds from the sale of my book is given to non-profit organizations. Recently, I established The Diana Dyer Cancer Survivors' Nutrition and Cancer Research Endowment Fund at The American Institute for Cancer Research in Washington, DC. This fund will provide money for research that will focus on defining nutrition strategies to optimize long-term survival after a cancer diagnosis.

After reading this book, if you believe you would have benefited by receiving it as educational material from your own cancer center, please tell someone there. The Registered Dietitian, the Clinical Nurse Specialist, the Education Coordinator, your Physician, and the Cancer Center Administrator would all be appropriate health care professionals with whom to share your request.

In this edition, I have done some updates, added an extensive chapter containing tips for eating away from home, and made the book and print size larger, thus easier to read. I hope you find both information and inspiration in my book so that your cancer recovery journey is easier than mine was.

With best wishes,
Diana Dyer

February 1999

❧ Preface to the 2002 Printing

It's been five years since I stapled the first edition of my book at Kinko's. Looking back to that time, I never would have guessed that my early efforts at writing about my own cancer recovery would have spread so far and that so many meaningful changes for cancer survivors would be happening.

Of most significance to me is that The American Institute for Cancer Research (AICR) has expanded their mission to include nutrition education and research for cancer survivors. They are committed to helping answer the questions about what foods may help reduce the risk of a cancer recurrence or a second newly diagnosed cancer. AICR has sponsored national conferences on this topic to raise national awareness of the urgency for increased research funding and staffing by Registered Dietitians in cancer centers in order to thoroughly address these unmet needs.

Proceeds from the sale of my books, including the Spanish translation of *A Dietitian's Cancer Story*, continue to fund my endowment established at AICR in 2000. The Diana Dyer Cancer Survivors' Nutrition and Cancer Research Endowment funds research projects to help define nutritional strategies after a cancer diagnosis, either during treatment or recovery, that will help enhance the odds for long-term survival. I have recently helped to fund my first project, which is very meaningful to me. Additional donations to my endowment are welcome; call AICR at 1-800-843-8114 for more information.

In addition, it has been gratifying to hear of so many cancer centers around the country that are now offering various complementary therapies to newly diagnosed cancer patients as means of helping them gain control over their disease. Strategies such as nutrition and cooking classes, meditation, creative and guided imagery, yoga, T'ai chi, Qi Gong, hypnotherapy, acupuncture, art, music and dance therapies, journaling and writing sessions, along with support groups are some of the many ways cancer centers are helping survivors heal physically, emotionally, and spiritually from the trauma of a cancer diagnosis. Ongoing research will provide data to show if these therapies also enhance the odds for long-term survival.

I have connected with so many of my readers since 1997. Reaching outside of myself and advocating for all of you has given me incredible energy. While much has been accomplished, there is still so much to do, particularly in the area of cancer prevention. I urge you all to work in your little corner of the world to bring about positive change in some area of importance to you. It is never too late, and no effort is too small. Only God knows how far the ripples from your efforts will reach! The results of all our efforts are a testimony to my belief in the power of "active hope" to change ourselves and also our world.

To your health, healing, and hope!
Diana Grant Dyer, MS, RD

March 2002

Preface to the 2010 Printing

At the beginning of 2009, a friend passed on some words of wisdom that were shared by one of her patients who had recently died after a long and courageous journey with cancer. These words, "If you have a dream, make it happen", were both a driving force and guiding light during this past year. My husband and I have wanted to have a small organic farm since the beginning of our marriage. However, we had put our dream on hold while life handed us other responsibilities and opportunities, speed bumps, pot-holes, and detours, plus plenty of fear about what could happen in the future.

With those inspirational words in mind, along with hours and hours of thoughtful discussions about goals, hopes, fears, and dreams for our future (however long or short it may be), we took a deep breath and decided 2009 was the year to put trust in our dreams and make them happen, at last. Thus, we have finally purchased a house with some acreage on land that was formerly farmed. It will take years of work in order to develop our farm to become what we envision it can be, however, we are taking on this life-long project with energy, enthusiasm, and joy. Slowly, slowly, we are bringing love, life, and beauty back to this home and land.

A cancer diagnosis provides the gift of a "wake-up call", the acute awareness that we should actively seek our dreams, sooner rather than later. I particularly like the following quotations by Henry David Thoreau about dreams and goals:

Do not worry if you have built your castles in the air.
They are where they should be.
Now put the foundations under them.

If one advances confidently in the direction of his dreams,
and endeavors to live the life which he has imagined,
he will meet with success unexpected in common hours.

Dreams are the touchstones of our character.

We must walk consciously only part way toward our goal,
and then leap in the dark to our success.

I hope my experiences as a cancer survivor, along with some information and inspiration in my book, will help you thrive as a cancer survivor so you can build the foundations under your own dreams and then have the courage and confidence to leap toward them.

Diana Grant Dyer, MS, RD
January 2010

⚘ INTRODUCTION

The idea for this book was born after one of those defining moments in my life. On April 8, 1997, The *Detroit Free Press* published an article entitled "Nutrition vs. Cancer" in which my recovery from a childhood cancer, neuroblastoma, and two separate breast cancers, at ages 34 and 45, was highlighted. In addition to providing an overview of current knowledge, guidelines, and research evaluating the nutrition and cancer connections, the article discussed the changes that I, as a Registered Dietitian, have made in my diet and lifestyle to minimize the risk of cancer recurrence after my second breast cancer. I did have a mastectomy and chemotherapy with each breast cancer. However, I have chosen to recover from my second breast cancer very differently from my first one by making significant changes in both my diet and lifestyle, many of which fall under the umbrella term of complementary and alternative medicine (CAM).

When the *Detroit Free Press'* medical writer, Pat Anstett, suggested my telephone number be included in the article, I could not foresee why she thought that would be necessary. However, my phone began ringing before 9:00 a.m. the morning the article was published and continued almost non-stop for months following the article's distribution to newspapers throughout the country over the Knight-Ridder wire service. Additionally, the article has been clipped and sent to friends and relatives from all sections of the U.S., Canada, and at least six other countries that I have been told about. Although most of the articles reprinted in other newspapers did not publish my telephone number, people were creative, found my number, and called. I now truly understand the power of the written word! And people are still calling several years later!

The responses to this article ranged from simple "Congratulations" to multiple requests for more information on the changes I have made in my diet and lifestyle. Cancer patients frequently ask of both their health care practitioner and themselves, "What else can I be doing to help fight my cancer, reduce my risks of a recurrence, or even keep a new cancer from developing?" Almost everyone who called asked me to write a book giving more information about my experiences, the changes I have made in my diet and lifestyle in order to address these important questions, and my resources.

A breast cancer survivor calling from New Jersey told me the unique combination of both my lengthy experience as a cancer patient and survivor in conjunction with my scientific training as a Registered Dietitian gave her confidence that I would not allow myself to be steered wrong about the choices I made for recovering from this latest cancer. She accurately summarized my approach to recovery this time. I tried diligently to simultaneously wear both my patient and clinician hats as I explored which conventional cancer therapy was right for me along with which alternative or complementary therapies might supplement and enhance (not replace) the conventional treatments for my most recent cancer.

I wrote this book to give those people interested in an integrated and comprehensive approach for optimizing health after cancer a jump start onto that path. It is precisely what I wish my own cancer center could have had available to give me when I asked, "What else can I be doing?" It gives the details of my own path and journey. It is a concise guidebook, not an overwhelming, detailed regimen, nor is it a tightly scheduled itinerary on a tour bus. You can pick and choose the strategies that appeal to you when you are ready to incorporate them into your life.

I wish you the very best for both optimal health and healing after your cancer diagnosis. Thank you all for your prayers, best wishes, and confidence in me.

MY CANCER STORY

I was diagnosed with neuroblastoma, a childhood cancer, when I was six months old in 1950. It was treated successfully with surgery plus very large doses of radiation therapy, and I had a normal, healthy childhood. However, my parents, and later I, were extra vigilant regarding my subsequent health, always wondering if any additional health problems might develop secondary to the radiation therapy that cured me of my first cancer. I first had two "cancer scares" developing a thyroid tumor in 1962 and ovarian tumors in 1972, both of which, thankfully, were benign. In 1981, I sought out the advice of an oncologist regarding my concerns about the potential for still developing any subsequent cancer. As he discussed what was known and what wasn't known yet about breast cancer risk following radiation at a young age, I remember thinking "Breast cancer is for 'old' women—I don't really need to worry about that yet." However, I did start doing monthly self-breast exams, which likely saved my life just three years later.

When I was 34 years old, I discovered a lump in my left breast, which had clearly not been there the month before. I had even had a breast exam by my physician three weeks earlier with no sign of a lump (and I remember commenting to him that I felt terrific!). Upon biopsy, the lump was determined to be malignant, an invasive intraductal carcinoma with indeterminate estrogen receptor status. Due to the large amount of radiation I received after my neuroblastoma diagnosis, a lumpectomy followed by radiation therapy was not an option for me. Therefore, I had a modified radical mastectomy with lymph node dissection, which showed one positive node. I underwent 6 cycles of chemotherapy (Cytoxan, Methotrexate, and 5-FU) and took the anti-estrogen drug Tamoxifen. After that time period was over, I submerged my fears about what might still come and coped by adopting the simple belief that this was now all behind me. I jumped back into my life, which centered on my husband, raising my two sons, ages seven and two, and developing my career.

My second breast cancer was first noticed as a suspicious area seen on my 10 year anniversary mammogram, and subsequently determined to be malignant after a biopsy. I was shocked and really angry this time—I couldn't believe it! My life was in full swing—I had no time slots open in my Franklin Planner™ for cancer again! And why was this still happening to me? I thought I had lived a very healthy lifestyle, and I also naively thought, "I've paid my dues" by having cancer twice already. This was a brand new cancer, not a recurrence. Therefore, while it seemed surgery and chemotherapy had cured me of my first breast cancer, just choosing those two modalities of treatment were obviously not enough to keep a new cancer from developing in me. Besides, even though my new tumor was small (1.4 cm), this cancer was much more advanced than my first breast cancer, having nine positive axillary lymph nodes and one positive deep intermammary lymph node found with a PET scan, putting me at very high risk for recurrence this time.

It was time to start looking at things in a new way. I never questioned that chemotherapy and surgery would play a role in my treatment with this second breast cancer. However, because of my apparent high risk factors from the radiation therapy and who knows what else, I now knew I could no longer naively think that chemotherapy and surgery alone were all I needed to do to keep this cancer from coming back or even another new one from developing.

I was finally ready to turn around in order to both confront and embrace my cancer history. In addition, I knew that it was finally time for me to go beyond coping (which I had obviously done very well for 45 years!) to healing—physically, emotionally, and spiritually. Although I was choosing a mastectomy and chemotherapy (Adriamycin and Cytoxan) as the first-line offense against my disease, I was determined to figure out what else I could do to enhance the long-term effectiveness of these treatments by identifying and changing various aspects of my lifestyle.

The challenge that I accepted for myself was to see if I could put together a healing recipe, looking for the best ingredients that conventional oncology therapy had to offer and complementing it with additional therapies from the uncharted world of alternative medicine and as such, see if I could tweak my fate.

I remember telling my husband after chemotherapy was completed that, as hard as the previous six months had been, I knew that the next six months were going to be even more difficult. The process of doing a life review and determining what aspects to change that might offer some hope for reducing my cancer odds was daunting. It was not a quick process, nor an easy one. I started by coming home from my last chemotherapy session thinking "Now what?" and feeling very alone, lost and abandoned. (Feeling abandoned by the medical system of which professionally I was a part was doubly difficult.) As I left my last chemo session, no one even told me good-bye or good luck. More importantly, I wish that someone would have handed me a little "map" or a guidebook describing the options I had for the multiple lifestyle changes that could be considered for their potential of both reducing my risks of recurrence and facilitating healing. I hope this book now serves as that map or guidebook for others.

I'm fully aware and accept that there are no guarantees for cancer recovery. Cancer is a disease that has baffled the best scientists, physicians, and healers over the ages, but I don't believe anyone will dispute there are lifestyle changes that can be done to tip the scales in a person's favor for both fighting the disease and achieving the optimal health possible. All the research studies aren't done, many of them haven't even been started yet, however, I didn't have time to wait for all the answers to be defined to the complete satisfaction of the scientific community before I made changes.

Therefore, I have tried to determine what is known, what's not, what's controversial, what's harmless to try, what's least expensive, what offers real hope compared to hype or even potential harm, and subsequently developed a healing recipe for myself. It is my belief that no one ingredient has been the magic bullet responsible for my healing. I also believe true healing does not have to be a cure and is only possible through a holistic, multi-faceted approach providing for my physical, emotional, mental, and spiritual needs. In addition, I don't believe there is only one right answer. Qi gong and soy shakes might be right for me, but yoga and various teas right for you.

I share with you my two favorite quotations:

- "I encourage my patients to have faith in God
  but not to expect Him (Her) to do all the work."
  —Dr. Bernie Siegel, *Love, Medicine, and Miracles*

- "When the dog is chasing you, turn around and whistle for it."
  —Henry David Thoreau

Both of them have been very inspirational to me, as I have stopped running from my cancer history and begun working toward recovering and healing after my latest cancer.

I am now well past my most recent diagnosis in 1995 and still considered cancer-free. It is amazing to me how much I have changed during this time. I have made many major lifestyle changes already, but I am still working on others. While I wouldn't wish cancer on anyone, I have a sense of accomplishment, satisfaction, and contentment with my life right now that wouldn't be there without my latest cancer experience. It is my hope that some aspect of this book will resonate with you and be helpful as you begin your journey toward recovery and healing after cancer.

NUTRITIONAL GUIDELINES TO REDUCE CANCER RISK

Why did I think I needed to change my diet? Wasn't I, as a dietitian, eating healthy before? Yes, I was. I had cut back to eating bratwurst only once each year, ate my "5-A-Day," cut my overall fat intake to 30 percent years ago, ate double cheese pizza and high fat yummy ice cream only in moderation—all the right things according to published guidelines to reduce cancer risk. Maybe eating as healthfully as I had been kept me from getting my two breast cancers sooner, maybe even helped keep me alive after my first one. However, if I, as a dietitian, believed that "we are what we eat," I felt compelled after my second breast cancer to accept the challenge of changing my food intake to create a biochemical environment in my body that was potentially less conducive to and/or more protective against cancer. I wanted everything I put in my mouth to truly help maximize my potential for long-term survival from cancer.

Research to understand the optimal diet to treat cancer, prevent cancer or a recurrence is still on-going and evolving. Many questions are still unanswered, particularly regarding how, when, what types, and amounts of dietary fats contribute to the development of cancer. The same questions are still not fully understood regarding the role soy might have in preventing cancer. However, it is reassuring to know there are over 200 studies reported in the scientific literature showing diets high in fruits and vegetables reduce the risk of many types of cancer. In fact, research is "mushrooming" in the new area of phytochemicals (non-nutrient components of plants) and the role of these compounds from our food in the prevention and treatment of cancer.

The American Cancer Society, The National Cancer Institute, and The American Institute for Cancer Research have published dietary guidelines based on multiple research studies. Knowing there are no guarantees, using these guidelines and other information in the scientific literature, I have created my own nutrition action plan to help minimize my risk of both recurrent breast cancer and even a potential brand new type of cancer. In addition, I devised this nutrition action plan to optimize my overall health by reducing the risk of developing the debilitating chronic diseases that are prevalent in this country plus can also develop secondary to some cancer therapies.

My own professional organizations might say I've unnecessarily taken my diet to a point that is not yet scientifically supported regarding my desire to reduce the risk of cancer recurrence. However, they would also say that my diet is nutritionally adequate, healthy, and not dangerous in any way. In fact, it was because my risk of recurrence was so high (and there are still so many loose ends with understanding the entire nutrition and cancer connection) that I created this diet for myself in order to address many of those still unanswered questions. I needed to personally draw a line in the sand on many controversial questions such as how much and what types of fat to include in my diet, how many and which types of fruits and vegetables to eat, organic vs. non-organic foods, how much soy (if any) to include. The questions go on and on.

I read extensively in the scientific nutritional literature to more clearly understand what was known, what was not, and what is considered controversial in the field of cancer and nutrition. I've spoken personally with many researchers to both make sure I was understanding their research and to see what their thoughts were regarding the diet plan I was developing for myself.

In addition, I worked hard in my own kitchen to see if this ultrahealthy diet was indeed "doable." Could a dietitian who had only tasted soymilk at a conference and never incorporated tofu into her family's diet do more than "talk the talk?" Could I actually "walk the walk?" I have done it, and you can, too. It is workable, tasty, and enjoyable, and, I have done it with a minimum of stress or obsession.

My family was a good sport about all my dietary changes and tried everything for the first six to nine months or so. At some point though, they politely put their collective foot down and said, "No more beans every night or tofu hot dogs!" So I began figuring out how to do this for me without cooking two complete meals (more time, more stress), and I have included some of my tips for that, too.

I had many difficulties tolerating my chemotherapy during which time I admittedly ate whatever I could. I did not fully implement this entire new nutrition plan until after I completed my chemo and was starting to regain my strength, lose my "chemo brain," and have my taste sensations begin to normalize. For those of you with a better tolerance to your chemo, I would strongly suggest implementing these changes as soon after your diagnosis as possible. In fact, I have heard from hundreds of people who have already bought this book that making these changes has been easier than they thought and also beneficial. Many, many people have called me or written to say my shake recipe "got them through chemo" and also helped them with full recovery by "energizing" them! So wherever you are in your cancer journey, it's never too early to start with changes, but it's not too late either. Every change you make is one step toward both improving your chances for long-term survival from cancer and your quality of life.

Don't feel overwhelmed though! It took me almost a year after I completed my chemotherapy to fully implement this plan for myself and still be able to feed my family, too! You'll be able to do it faster because I was researching at the same time. So, start by making a goal of experimenting and changing one component per month in your diet. Start by changing what seems easiest to you. Maybe that will be making my shake every day. Next you might try to consistently incorporate nine+ servings of fruits and veggies into your daily diet. Every little change is potentially helpful, and any change is better than none. You can do it!

The following components of my diet plan are listed in order of importance to me personally, and also, as I best understand the strength of the scientific evidence for their role in the nutrition and cancer connection.

A word about Diana's diet plan:

The following information consists of general guidelines. You may have a medical condition for which additional modification of these guidelines would be appropriate. Please discuss any planned changes with your health care professionals. Every cancer center should have a Registered Dietitian (RD) on its staff available to assess your nutritional requirements and make specific suggestions, ideally, an RD with an additional specialty certification in oncology nutrition (CSO). If a dietitian is not available at your cancer center, or the staffing is inadequate, please advocate for increased accessibility to an RD at your cancer center so nutrition services can be available in a pro-active, in-depth, and individualized manner. Don't wait until you have lost or gained a significant amount of weight to see a dietitian for information to help you.

Nutritional Components

❦ Prepare and eat all meals in a loving, caring manner. The fast food era of our life is a thing of the past. This has required a major life-style change to which I am committed. I can't tell you how to do this for your own family, but it was the most important thing for me. We eat sit-down meals without the TV or dashing somewhere almost every night of the week. I do think of the time I spend fixing meals everyday as a necessary ingredient in my total healing recipe.

A Dietitian's Cancer Story

🍎 Achieve and maintain a healthy weight for your height. Regular exercise is very important both to optimize health, achieve a healthy weight, and maximize the function of our immune system. When I really forced myself to examine how frequently I exercised prior to this latest cancer, I had to admit I exercised whenever I could. I was not faithful. I now briskly walk/run two to three miles five to seven days per week and have begun strength training three times per week.

🍎 Eliminate/reduce alcohol intake. This was not hard for me to change. When I do occasionally have a drink, I choose a red wine or a dark beer, both of which have higher phytochemical contents than white wine or regular beer.

🍎 Increase fiber to 25 to 30 grams per day. The average American intake is 10 to 12 grams per day, and I was not above average before. Wow, was that hard to admit!

- Three to six servings per day of whole grain foods (more than six if higher calories needed)

- One to two servings per day of beans, legumes, and nuts

- Five to nine+ servings per day of fruits and vegetables, at least three different colors each day

A fiber intake of this amount is very easy to achieve when your diet is based on fruits, vegetables and whole grains, beans, legumes, and nuts. I now have a personal goal of a minimum of nine servings of fruits and vegetables each day. I aim for three servings at each meal plus snacks of fruits or vegetables each day. The darkest colored fruits and vegetables have the highest content of phytochemicals. Toss out your iceberg lettuce and use spinach, kale, romaine, leaf lettuce, or other greens instead.

You may need to increase fiber gradually to minimize GI distress. Use of a product like Beano® from your drug store will help cut down gas production from legumes until your body adapts to a regular intake. I always have some beans and legumes cooked and in the refrig or freezer to use. I also use a lot of canned cooked beans since they are so fast and easy to keep on the pantry shelf. As you increase fiber, be sure to increase your fluid intake, too.

🍎 Reduce fat in your diet to approximately 20 percent of your caloric intake.

- 16 to 18 percent fat in our diet is the minimum amount required in order to maximize the absorption of the fat-soluble (cancer-fighting) phytochemicals (*source:* C. Rock, PhD, RD). It's not known yet if the very low fat diets (10 percent or less) designed for reversing heart disease can also maximize one's cancer reduction potential. This is where identifying your medical and nutritional priorities is important and individualizing a diet plan can best be done with the guidance of a Registered Dietitian.

- Consume a small amount of fat with between-meal fruit and vegetable snacks to ensure maximum absorption of the phyto- chemicals. Most of the phytochemicals are fat-soluble like beta-carotene and Vitamin A and need some fat eaten with them to get the highest quantity possible absorbed and into the blood stream so they can do their cancer-fighting action in your body's cells. I eat a small amount of soynut butter (like peanut butter), soy nuts (easy to carry in my purse and/or brief case), nuts, pine nuts, or hummus along with my between meal fruit and veggie snacks.

- Use only extra-virgin olive oil or canola oil in your regular cooking.

- Eliminate regular margarines, liquid corn oil and other veg- etable/seed oils from regular use. Olive and canola oils are high- est in monounsaturated fats that may confer protection against cancer. I do use a small amount of dark sesame oil for flavoring Asian recipes. Using my blender, I combine butter and olive oil into a spread for fresh bread (I use only very small amounts of this). Additionally, there are a few margarine products entering the market that are free of trans-fatty acids, which are the hydrogenated, or partially-hardened, polyunsaturated fats that may also contribute to increased cancer risk. (Other sources of these potentially harmful trans-fatty acids are many commer- cially prepared bakery goods, crackers, and snack foods.)

- Example: for an intake of 1,600-1,800-2,000 calories per day, a 20 percent fat diet would equal 36-40-44 grams of fat per day. You have to read food labels and be honest about serving sizes that you are eating. Have a dietitian help you figure your approx- imate caloric needs and resulting range of fat intake to consume.

♦ Buy only very lean meats, eat processed meats (like lunch meats, etc.) only very rarely if you consume meats at all, and reduce portion size to two to three ounces per meal (approximately the size of a deck of play- ing cards). Think of meats as an accent for the other food items on a plate instead of the main attraction. Consider purchasing meats and poultry grown without the use of hormones, antibiotics, and those that have been grass-fed, pasture-raised, or fed organic feed.

♦ Use reduced-fat (not no-fat) dairy products, consuming one to three servings per day. Dairy fat has the highest concentration of a molecule called "conjugated linoleic acid" or "CLA" for short, which has demonstrated anti-cancer activity in the laboratory. CLA is present in higher concentration in organic milk products when dairy cows are grass-fed. Another reason to consider using dairy products from non-BST (growth hormone) treated cows is they contain lower levels of a molecule called Insulin-like Growth Factor (IGF-1). Higher blood levels of IGF-1 have been associated with several types of cancer, and obesity may turn out to be the main reason for higher IGF-1 blood levels. Much more research needs to be completed to clarify the relationship between IGF-1 and cancer, but in the meantime, I consider this a loose end and prefer to eliminate this possible risk factor from my diet. I now use only pasteurized organic dairy products from non-BST treated cows that have been primarily grass (not grain) fed. I can buy many products in my regular grocery store, but others I get at a health food store. Dairy products are a good source of calcium, plus low-fat dairy foods (milk, yogurt, and cheese) have been associated with decreased risk for colon cancer and breast cancer.

♣ Consume soy food products one to three servings/day. Soybeans have many anti-carcinogenic compounds, some of which (the phytoestrogen genistein) are unique to soybeans. We do not yet know the exact amount of soy to consume in our diet, or even at which age, for a protective effect. We also don't know which cancers may be prevented by soy or possibly benefit from soy consumption as part of treatment. We also don't know if soy will be able to confer any protection or benefits if one continues to eat a high fat diet low in plant foods.

However current research shows that even as little as one serving each day may offer some advantage to reducing cancer risk. Similar to a traditional Japanese diet, I eat one to three servings of soy foods daily, primarily using soymilk, tofu, tempeh, soybeans, soynut butter, soy flour, and miso. Not all soy foods currently have all of the important cancer fighting compounds due to the processing of the soy protein. Products made from isolated soy protein will contain more of the phytoestrogens (also called isoflavones) than products made with concentrated soy protein. Be sure to read food labels. Some companies are even starting to add the isoflavone content of their product on the labels.

I recommend focusing on introducing soy foods, rather than supplements, into a diet in order to take advantage of the multiple anti-carcinogenic properties that whole soy foods potentially have to offer. When available, I purchase foods made from organic soybeans that have been grown in the United States instead of imported. Don't go overboard though. Eating a pound of tofu every day may be potentially harmful due to large amount of phytoestrogens. Currently, confusion and controversy surround the inclusion of soy products for those people with cancers that are hormone-responsive. An example would be a woman with ER+, post-menopausal breast cancer, being treated with the anti-estrogen drug Tamoxifen. (I myself fit this profile.)

Do the phytoestrogens in soy "fuel" cancer growth for this type of cancer? Do they compete with and make the Tamoxifen less effective? Do they possibly even enhance Tamoxifen's benefits? Are they neutral or are they even beneficial for reducing cancer risk in their own right? I follow this research very closely and post relevant information on my website. In addition, I recommend that you consult with your oncologist and/or dietitian for the latest research results in this area of study. However, I have been consuming one to three servings of organic soy foods on a daily basis since 1995 without a recurrence. (See FAQ #11 on page 91 and FAQ #15 on page 98 for further discussion of this concern.)

🍎 Consume cold water fish two to three times per week (approximately one pound per week). Salmon, mackerel, white tuna, sardines, bluefish, ocean trout, and herring are all high in the omega-3 fatty acids that may help fight cancer. Of these, I prefer salmon and tuna and make an effort to eat approximately one pound total each week. Almost all restaurants have salmon on the menu now which makes it easier to go out to eat. Fortunately my whole family loves seafood, so two meals each week are easy to fix for all of us to eat the same food together. (See FAQ #10 on page 90 for additional information about purchasing seafood.)

🍎 Limit grilled, broiled, "blackened" meats and fish to special occasions only. This type of cooking, unfortunately, produces carcinogens. Steamed, microwaved, baked, boiled, poached, or stewed food preparation is healthier. (Grilling veggies does not produce the same carcinogens.) Marinating meats prior to grilling and turning meats approximately each minute while grilling does greatly reduce the carcinogens produced.

🍎 Liberally make use of various herbs and spices in your cooking for both enhancing flavor with low fat foods and increasing your intake of phytochemicals that may have a role in fighting cancer. Use a wide variety. (See page 45 for a list of culinary herbs with anti-cancer activity.)

🍎 Flaxseeds, ground flaxseed meal, and flaxseed oil are a plant source of an omega-3 fatty acid (alpha-linolenic acid or ALA) that may be valuable to help fight cancer. In addition, flaxseeds, but not the oil, are the most concentrated plant source of a phytochemical called lignan that bacteria in our large bowel convert to a molecule with anti-estrogen properties which may be useful in preventing or treating tumors that are estrogen responsive. I use one to two tablespoons of ground flaxseed meal per day. The optimal amount to include in our diets to prevent or treat cancer, and which cancers, is the subject of much current research.

What Counts as a Serving Size?

- Meats :
  - 2 to 3 oz. of cooked lean meat, poultry or fish (about the size of a deck of cards)

- Dairy Foods and Eggs:
  - 1 cup milk or yogurt
  - 2 ounces processed cheese
  - 1-1/2 oz. natural cheese
  - 1 egg

- Grains:
  - 1 slice of bread, 1/2 bagel, 1 dinner roll
  - 1 ounce ready to eat cereal
  - 1/2 cup cooked cereal, rice or pasta

- Beans and Nuts:
  - 1/2 cup cooked dry beans
  - 1/3 cup nuts
  - 2 Tbsp. peanut butter

- Fruit:
  - 1 medium apple, banana or orange
  - 3/4 cup fruit juice
  - 1/2 cup chopped, cooked, or canned fruit
  - 1/4 cup dried fruit

- Vegetables:
  - 1 cup raw leafy vegetables
  - 3/4 cup vegetable juice
  - 1/2 cup other cooked or raw vegetables, chopped

- Soy products:
  - 1 cup soy milk
  - 1/2 cup tempeh
  - 1/4 cup soy butter
  - 1/2 cup (4 oz.) tofu
  - 2 tablespoons soy nuts

How to Achieve Nine+ Servings/Day of Fruits and Vegetables without Chomping Carrots All Day Long!

As a dietitian, I knew I was eating my "5-A-Day" quite consistently. I made a new goal to consume a minimum of nine servings daily to better provide my body's biochemistry with the cancer-fighting phytochemicals. I wanted to do that by eating whole foods, but I had trouble imagining how I would eat more! I've found it's actually not that hard to do, but it does take thought and planning. It doesn't happen by accident. Here are some helpful suggestions:

🍎 My soy shake recipes on pages 38 to 39 each contain three servings of fruit and veggies. That is my breakfast each morning. I can't drink it all right away, so what I don't finish at breakfast, I put into an insulated coffee mug with a lid and a straw and drink over the next hour or so.

🍎 Fresh or dried fruit for between meal snacks. I keep dried fruit in a plastic bag inside my briefcase. I also will throw in an apple or banana.

🍎 Drink 100 percent juices. I prefer juices packed with phytochemicals such as orange, carrot, and tomato or mixed vegetable juices.

🍎 Make up large amounts of tossed salad with lots of extra veggies cut up in them so you are getting a variety. Also, that way you've already got a salad ready for tomorrow's lunch or supper. I use the new vegetable storage plastic bags to help keep all the veggies fresh.

🍎 Add fruit to salads like apples, mandarin oranges, dried cranberries or cherries.

🍎 Mix fruit with plain yogurt for a snack.

🍎 Cut up an assortment of veggies to be readily available for snacks. I often have red pepper strips with hummus for an afternoon snack.

🍎 Add extra vegetables to soup, either homemade or canned.

🍎 Decrease or even eliminate the meat and cheese in a sandwich and increase the veggies—extra lettuce, tomato, broccoli sprouts, pepper strips, avocado.

🍎 Buy tabouli already made in the deli section of your grocery store for a quick and easy source of numerous phytochemicals.

🍎 Load up with lots of raw veggies at the salad bar. Use dark lettuce and spinach—not icberg.

🍎 Make kebobs for the grill that are veggies and fruit with zucchini, yellow squash, onion, mushrooms, cherry tomatoes, sweet peppers, eggplant, pineapple wedges, peach slices, etc.

🍎 Thawed frozen fruit on top of angel food cake makes a nice dessert.

✦ Keep a small box of raisins in your desk at work, briefcase, or the car.

✦ Make low fat quiche with veggies. I use up leftover veggies this way.

✦ Keep plenty of salsa on hand as a dip for veggies or low-fat chips.

✦ Try a new fruit or veggie each week. Some grocery stores now have dietitians working for them now to help you with cooking ideas. At the very least, the stores will have recipe cards to guide you with something new.

✦ Buy small snack-packs of canned fruit to take for lunch.

✦ Mix last night's left over veggies into tonight's salad.

✦ When you're baking anything, throw into the oven some potatoes, sweet potatoes, and winter squash for that day or later in the week to reheat in the microwave when you have less time.

✦ Have a baked potato and juice at a fast food restaurant. Top the potato with salsa.

✦ Look for already peeled, sliced, or even shredded fruits and/or vegetables at the grocery store for ultimate convenience.

✦ Put extra veggies into spaghetti sauce. Shredded carrots are nice.

✦ We serve stir-fried veggies once every week. We vary the meat and veggie (I use tofu, tempeh, or simply some beans with mine).

✦ Make a veggie pizza with lots of broccoli, mushrooms, peppers, artichoke hearts, onions, dried tomatoes, olives.

✦ Make reduced-fat fruit desserts like baked apples, crisps, and cobblers.

Even my family regularly eats six to nine servings per day of fruits and vegetables now. Be creative and give it a try. You'll be surprised. It's easier than you think!

Sample Menu:

✦ Breakfast
   • My shake. One day I might use mangos and raspberries for the fruit ingredients and another day I might use only blueberries. Experiment. Sometimes I even use leftover sweet potatoes instead of the carrots. I use a brand of soymilk that is highest in protein and fortified with calcium. (See my grocery list in the Appendix.)

❖ Morning Snack
  • 3/4 cup of pink grapefruit juice (higher in phytochemicals than plain)
  • four to five low-fat, high-fiber crackers

❖ Lunch
  • Dehydrated bean soup in one of those cardboard containers (look for one that is highest in protein and fiber and lowest in sodium) or homemade soup, left-over veggie-type casserole
  • Whole-grain bagel
  • 1/2 pink grapefruit
  • 1/2 sweet red pepper cut into strips with some hummus for dip
  • one 8 oz. carton fruit/veggie juice

❖ Afternoon snack
  • five to six dried apricots
  • four to five almonds

❖ Supper
  • I might cook my family baked chicken with crispy bread-crumbs according to a Jane Brody recipe. For myself, I would bake a couple slices of extra-firm tofu coated with the bread crumb mixture, too, right along with the chicken.
  • one cup instant brown rice
  • one cup steamed fresh or frozen broccoli
  • one cup tossed salad with romaine lettuce, kale, and other veggies
  • one cup 1 percent milk

I use one to two teaspoons of olive oil and a flavored vinegar for dressing on my salad. I also would put about one teaspoon of the butter/olive oil spread on my broccoli for extra flavor and also to get the fat amount up to 20 percent of the diet.

❖ PM Snack
  • eight oz. low-fat yogurt
  • 1/2 apple with one teaspoon soy butter
  • Decaffeinated tea of various kinds

This is just one sample menu. It contains approximately 2000 calories, 45 grams of fat (20 percent), 12 servings of fruits and vegetables. Five to six servings of whole grains (I count the fiber I get from the wheat bran and wheat germ in the shake, too), two to three servings of soy, one serving of legumes, two dairy products, plenty of high quality protein from the dairy, legumes, and soy products, and overall, a very balanced and healthful diet.

Additional Tips for Integrating this Diet with a Family

 It's only the entree that I have to think about. Everything else is the same.

 Fortunately, my family loves seafood of any kind, so we regularly have two seafood meals each week.

 We have stir-fry once each week, always varying the vegetables and the meats. It's easy to make this both with and without added meat. For myself, I might add tofu, tempeh, seitan (a wheat gluten product), or beans.

 The veggie burgers come in handy when my family wants burgers. I would even make one for myself if they were having something like pork chops.

 There are meat substitutes for bacon, sausage, hot dogs, bratwurst, chicken nuggets, etc. I use those only once in a while when needed as a substitute for the real thing for me.

 Tacos, burritos, fajitas are all easy. I can make mine with just beans at the same time I'm making theirs.

 I use the frozen textured vegetable protein that looks and cooks just like cooked ground hamburger for spaghetti sauce, chili, sloppy joes, etc.

 If I'm making a recipe that has a sauce of any kind, I just substitute tofu for the meat, like in chicken cacciatorie, in a separate pan or baking dish for me.

 If we order delivery pizza, I have enough time to make my own using whole wheat pizza crust or pita bread, tomato sauce, fresh veggies, and tofu or reduced-fat mozzarella cheese.

 My Web site (www.CancerRD.com) contains two weeks of family-tested, easy and tasty menus, complete with recipes, that follow my complete nutrition plan. I am always adding new recipes to my Web site, too, so keep checking back often.

🦢 DIANA'S GROCERY LIST

The following food items are those that I try to keep on hand at all times. Where specific brand names are mentioned, it is because I have found myself buying those products consistently for their taste and nutritional qualities. Your section of the country will likely have other or additional brands that are very good. Brands also sometimes change their contents, so I have learned to always check labels.

My husband and I grow a large portion of our own organic vegetables (see the section Gardening on pages 72 to 74.) I do most of my additional shopping at Farmers' Markets, regular grocery stores, going to natural food or health food stores one to two times each month. My family eats most of this food (not all) and I do buy other healthy foods (and treats, too) for them. My husband and I cook most of our food from scratch (we use very few convenience or processed food items), and we purchase as much organic and locally-grown food items as possible, when they are available and affordable.

Produce Section:

Apples
Apricots (dried)
Avocados
Bananas
Berries—any kind
Broccoli
Broccoli Sprouts—*wash very thoroughly and avoid if immune-compromised*
Cabbage—red
Carrots—baby and regular
Cauliflower
Cherries (dried)
Craisins
Garlic
Ginger (fresh)
Grapes (red)
Grapefruit (red)
Green Onions
Kale and other greens like chard
Melons—any kind
Onions
Oranges
Prunes
Raisins

Romaine Lettuce and baby lettuces
Shiitake Mushrooms
Spinach
Sweet Peppers (red, yellow, and orange)
Sweet Potatoes
Tofu, soft and firm—organic and non-GMO
Watercress
Winter Squash

My Grocery Store's "Health Food Section"

Baked soy squares—various flavors (White Wave)—
    in the refrigerator section
Boca Bratwurst®
Boca Burgers®—veggie burgers in the freezer section
Bulgur—(Bob's Red Mill ™)—on the shelf
Chips—baked by Guiltless Gourmet
Dried bean soups (Health Valley)—on the shelf
Eden® canned beans—look for black soybeans
Eden® pasta—look for 50-50 white/whole wheat
Hummus—in the deli section
Millet—(Bob's Red Mill™)—on the shelf
Rice—organic by Lundberg Farms
Silken tofu, vacuum-packed (Mori-Nu)—on the shelf
Soy cheese—mozzarella and cheddar—in the refrigerator section
Soy Milk—look for USDA organic on the label
Tabouli—in the deli section
Tempeh (White Wave)—in the refrigerator section
Tofu dogs—in the refrigerator section
Vruit™ (100 percent fruit/veggie juice)—three-pack—on the shelf
Whole wheat cous-cous (Fantastic Foods)—on the shelf

Seafood/Meats

Salmon filets or steaks
Tuna filets or steaks

Canned Goods

Applesauce, unsweetened
Artichoke hearts, in water
Beans, all varieties
Bean soups
Black olives
Canola Oil—cold expellor pressed
Extra Virgin olive oil

Prunes, pureed—baby food
Salmon
Tuna—Albacore in water (look for highest fat content per serving)

Dry Goods and other Miscellaneous Items

All-Bran® cereal
Brown rice, instant
Brownberry®—Whole Wheat and Health Nut bagels
Dried beans
Green tea
Kashi®—The Breakfast Pilaf
Low-fat spaghetti sauce
Rolled oats—original, or quick (not instant)
Salsa
Triscuits®—low-fat
Wasa® Fiber Rye crackers
Whole wheat pita bread
Whole wheat flat bread
Whole wheat bread

Frozen Foods

Egg Substitutes
Freshlike® Baby Broccoli Blend—featuring Sweet Beans® (green soybeans)
Frozen Fruit, unsweetened
Frozen veggies
Green Giant® Harvest Burgers® for Recipes™
Green Giant® Breakfast Links—Sausage Style
Morningstar Farms®
    Breakfast Strips - bacon style
    Chik Nuggets™
    Spicy Black Bean Burgers
Orange juice—w/calcium

Dairy Section

Eggs—Eggland's Best
Organic 1 percent Milk
Red/Pink Grapefruit Juice

Specialty Food Store

Better than Bouillon™ soup base
Olive-It® - butter and olive oil spread

A Dietitian's Cancer Story

Large Chain Natural Foods Store

Many of these items are now available in larger grocery stores:

Baked tofu squares—various flavors
Bread and bagels—by Natural Ovens
Miso
Organic butter
Organic cream cheese
Organic eggs
Organic feta cheese
Organic milk—both liquid and dry powder
Organic yogurt—lowfat by Stonyfield Farms™
Roasted SoyButter™ (like peanut butter) by Natural Touch®
Soy flour
Soy nuts
Spices—bulk
Tahini
Wheat bran—bulk
Wheat germ—bulk
Whole flaxseeds—bulk
Whole wheat pizza crusts (Kabuli brand)
Tempeh—various flavors

Feel free to photocopy this list for your own personal use. Tape it onto your refrigerator to mark those items you use up then take it with you to the grocery store.

DIANA'S "SUPERSOY & PHYTOCHEMICAL SHAKES"

I developed these shake recipes to provide beneficial phytochemicals (non-nutrient plant molecules) that are now thought to have multiple cancer-fighting activities. The shakes are all easy to prepare, consume, and digest. There are more than 1,000 phytochemicals in our foods from fruits, vegetables, whole grains, soy foods and other legumes. I drink one entire shake for breakfast daily. I consider it the centerpiece of my diet plan. It could also be consumed between meals. Many people have called or written me to say how tasty the shakes are and additionally, how helpful they have been with "getting through chemo" and "energizing" them. Drink to your health and enjoy!

The contents of a full recipe contain three servings from the fruit and vegetable groups, approximately 1-1/2 servings of soy, 40 to 60 percent of your daily calcium requirement, 33 to 40 percent of your daily fiber requirement, and a healthy dose of phytochemicals too numerous to count!

Recipe number one is completely lactose free, which is beneficial for those people that are lactose intolerant either prior to or temporarily during cancer therapy. Recipes number two through four are low in lactose and also, contain active bacterial cultures from the yogurt, which help maintain healthy, normal intestinal flora and may also help reduce cancer.

> **Special Notes regarding Diana's Shake Recipes:**
>
> ***Prostate cancer***—Data suggests there is an association between a high calcium intake and an increased risk of prostate cancer. A biological mechanism to explain these findings is emerging. Therefore, I recommend that men making the shake recipes for daily consumption use tofu and orange juice that are not calcium-fortified.
>
> ***Ovarian cancer***—Some data, but not all, show an increased risk of some types of ovarian cancer with increasing intake of milk and milk products. This possible relationship is not proven, but is what I call a "loose end". Therefore, I think it would be prudent for women with a family history of ovarian cancer to not consume the yogurt-containing shake recipes on a daily basis.

RECIPE #1

2-1/2 oz. soft tofu (cut a one pound block of tofu into six pieces)
6-8 baby carrots or one large carrot
3/4 cup fresh or frozen unsweetened fruit
1 Tbsp. wheat bran
1 Tbsp. wheat germ
1 Tbsp. whole flaxseed or ground flaxseed meal
3/4-cup soymilk (calcium fortified)
3/4 cup orange juice

Put ingredients into a blender. Start blender on a lower speed, then increase to high for one to three minutes to fully blend ingredients (variable time depending on blender's motor strength).

Makes about 3 cups. Approximate nutritional content:
Calories: 382 kcal   Protein: 18 gm   Fat: 8 gm
Carbohydrate: 60 gm   Fiber: 14 gm
Calcium: 430 mg (using calcium-fortified soy milk)

RECIPE #2

6-8 baby carrots or one large carrot
3/4 cup fresh or frozen unsweetened fruit
3 Tbsp. frozen juice concentrate (not diluted)
2-1/2 oz. tofu (cut a one pound block of tofu into six pieces)
1-cup soymilk
1 cup low-fat plain yogurt
1 Tbsp. wheat germ
1 Tbsp. wheat bran
1 Tbsp. whole flaxseeds or ground flaxseed meal

Makes about 4 cups. Approximate nutritional content:
Calories: 563 kcal   Protein: 30 gm   Fat: 11 gm
Carbohydrate: 78 gm   Fiber: 18 gm   Calcium: 604 mg

RECIPE #3

8 oz. (1 cup) soymilk
8 oz. (1 cup) vanilla low-fat yogurt
6-8 baby carrots or one large carrot
1/2 cup fresh fruit (mango is nice)
3/4 cup frozen fruit (raspberries make a pretty shake)
1 Tbsp. wheat germ
1 Tbsp. wheat bran
1 Tbsp. whole flaxseeds or ground flaxseed meal
2-1/2 oz. tofu (cut a one pound block of tofu into six pieces)

Makes about 4 cups. Approximate nutritional content:

Calories: 548 kcal	Protein: 27 gm	Fat: 12 gm
Carbohydrate: 84 gm	Fiber: 22 gm	Calcium: 625 mg

RECIPE #4

3/4 cup orange juice
8 oz. (1 cup) low-fat plain yogurt
4-oz. tofu (cut a one pound block of tofu into four equal pieces)
6-8 baby carrots or 1 large carrot
3/4 cup frozen unsweetened fruit
1 Tbsp. wheat germ
1 Tbsp. wheat bran
1 Tbsp. whole flaxseeds or ground flaxseed meal

Makes about 3 cups. Approximate nutritional content:

Calories: 465 kcal	Protein: 25 gm	Fat: 9 gm
Carbohydrate: 79 gm	Fiber: 18 gm	Calcium: 665 mg

Additional Helpful Hints:

❤ Look for tofu in the produce section of the grocery store. It should be kept cool.

❤ Change the tofu water daily.

❤ If you are severely immune-suppressed during or after your cancer therapy, you must minimize your risk of foodborne illness. Ask the Registered Dietitian where you receive your cancer treatments for guidelines of foods to avoid.

❤ I maximize my calcium intake by using a brand of tofu with calcium sulfate or gypsum, not nigari, and also calcium-fortified orange juice and soymilk.

❤ Buying both wheat bran and wheat germ in bulk at a health food store is much cheaper.

❤ Choose a brand of soy milk that is highest in protein.

❤ If an even less sweet shake is more appealing (especially while you are on chemo), add frozen cranberries as part of the fruit.

❤ Buy whole flaxseeds at a health food store. To make your own flax meal, grind about 1/2 cup in a blender for a few seconds, then store both seeds and the ground meal in the freezer.

❤ Buy yogurt that contains active, live bacterial cultures.

❤ If you have mouth sores during cancer therapy, do not choose fruits that contain tiny seeds (such as blackberries) which can be irritating. Choose fruit or fruit juice that is non-acidic. Some cancer patients say that yogurt and buttermilk are both soothing and speed healing of mouth sores. Buttermilk could be substituted for yogurt in any of the shakes.

❤ Start with small amounts of wheat germ, bran, and flax. Then gradually increase to the full amount. Be sure to drink lots of non-caffeinated fluids as you increase your fiber intake.

❤ Shake recipes two through four contain 690 to 750 mg calcium per entire shake recipe. Research now shows that approximately 500 mg calcium is the maximum amount that can be absorbed at one time. Thus, if you drink an entire shake in a short period of time (approximately 10 to 30 minutes), I would suggest using non-calcium-fortified juice or tofu. However, if you are likely to drink the shake much more slowly, over one to two hours like I do, then I still recommend using the calcium-fortified ingredients.

NUTRITION AND CANCER FATIGUE SUGGESTIONS

❦ Give yourself permission to rest with breaks and naps whenever you need to.

❦ Exercise with some moderate or gentle movements everyday. (Examples: walking, swimming, yoga, Tai Chi, Qi Gong are some suggestions)

❦ All treatment and disease side effects can contribute to fatigue. Tell your doctors about these symptoms so they can be treated aggressively with medical management if needed and/or complementary strategies. (Examples: nausea, vomiting, diarrhea, pain, shortness of breath, anxiety, depression, sleep difficulty, fevers, anorexia)

❦ Your doctor can also evaluate if there are any additional medical reasons why you might be fatigued.

❦ Eat a well balanced diet with enough calories and protein.

❦ Make every bite count—choose nutrient dense foods and beverages.

❦ Use a stool in the kitchen while preparing meals (I used one in the shower, too).

❦ Simplify, prioritize, and delegate everything you can (my friends lovingly prepared supper for my family for six straight months). Give your friends recipes to prepare.

❦ Keep foods handy that are quick and easy to prepare. Small snacks between meals can help you achieve an adequate intake of protein and calories.

❦ If the fatigue is overwhelming, keep high calorie and high protein snacks in a small cooler by your sofa or bed. (Note: This suggestion has a downside to it though because it is imperative to get up and move around frequently during the day to prevent other complications.)

❦ On days that you are feeling good, cook large batches of food and put the extra portions in the freezer.

❦ Eat your largest meal whenever you have the most energy during the day.

❦ Check to see if you qualify for Meals-on-Wheels service.

✦ If your food intake is inadequate, a multi-vitamin and mineral tablet may be appropriate. Check with the dietitian at your cancer center and your doctor.

✦ If you are having trouble consuming adequate calories and/or protein, a liquid supplement might help. Commercial products are available. Or make your own healthy shake using a recipe like "Diana's SuperSoy and Phytochemical Shake".

ADDITIONAL INFORMATION ABOUT FRUITS & VEGETABLES

People often ask me which fruits and vegetables are the best for preventing or fighting cancer. It is difficult to answer that question briefly because there are so many factors to consider. There is some research that has determined in the laboratory (test tube) which fruits and vegetables have the highest anti-oxidant activity, coming from the combined anti-oxidant activity of vitamins, minerals, and numerous phytochemicals. The following produce have the highest antioxidant activity in order of potency: (*Source:* J. Agri. Food Chem. 44:701, 3426, 1996)

🍎 Vegetables: kale, beets, red peppers, broccoli, spinach, potato, sweet potato, and corn

🍎 Fruits: blueberries and strawberries

The following have progressively lower levels:

🍎 Vegetables: cauliflower, egg-plant, carrots, string beans, cabbage, squash, garlic, iceberg lettuce, celery, onion, leaf lettuce, and cucumber

> On-going research will always show variations to this "order of importance". The bottom-line recommendation: Increase your intake from a wide-variety of fruit and vegetables on a daily basis.

🍎 Fruits: plums, oranges, red grapes, kiwi, pink grapefruit, white grapefruit, white grapes, apples, tomatoes, bananas, pears, and melons

Additional research will need to be done to validate factors regarding actual absorption of all of the phytochemicals and their impact on various metabolic activities in vivo (in real life situations—animal and human). Remember also that fruits and vegetables are important for more than their anti-oxidant capacity. Eat a wide variety of them for the hundreds, if not thousands, of phytochemicals they contain that have anti-cancer activity. Stay tuned in to this very exciting area.

All produce should be washed very thoroughly (including organically raised produce), especially types for which the outside rind or peel is not eaten, as a knife slicing through the item could drag bacteria or other microbial contaminants onto the part you consume potentially causing a foodborne illness. This is especially important if you are still immune-suppressed. In addition, washing by scrubbing with a vegetable brush when possible or soaking in water containing a teaspoon of dish detergent/gallon of water will help reduce pesticide content on produce that cannot be scrubbed. I would not recommend eating any type of sprouts if you are still immune-suppressed.

The question of pesticides always comes up. I do agree with those who believe we derive more health benefits from eating fruits and vegetables with pesticides than from not eating fruits and vegetables. There are more than 200 studies in the scientific literature that clearly show decreased risk for many chronic diseases, including cancer, with an increased consumption of fruits and vegetables. However, I consider the issue of pesticides and their potential harmful health effects a loose end.

The 12 Most Contaminated Fruits & Vegetables (2009 List)

- Peach
- Apple
- Bell Pepper
- Celery
- Nectarine
- Strawberry
- Cherries
- Kale
- Lettuce
- Grapes (imported)
- Carrot
- Pear

So, I have chosen to eat primarily organic produce, using published data analyses in which fruits and vegetables were analyzed and then ranked for their content of the most potentially risky pesticides. The Environmental Working Group (www.ewg.org), a consumer-based group based in Washington, DC, has analyzed FDA pesticide inspection data to rate fruits and vegetables as "The Dirty Dozen" and also "The Clean 15", publishing this information on its Web site. I do not let this controversy drive me crazy but use the information to make informed choices about which produce to buy and eat.

CULINARY HERBS & SPICES WITH ANTI-CANCER ACTIVITY

Don't forget that culinary herbs and spices may also help with the cancer prevention and cancer fighting process. Many herbs and spices commonly used in cooking are receiving increased attention and research as their components and actions in the body are more fully understood. These herbs and spices contain various substances (phytochemicals) that exert their anti-cancer actions by protecting cell structures as antioxidants, by blocking various hormone actions and metabolic pathways associated with the development of cancer, or they induce enzymes that help metabolize and eliminate carcinogens.

The following herbs and spices have the highest level of anti-cancer actions: garlic, ginger, licorice root, umbelliferous (carrot) family: anise, caraway, celery, chervil, cilantro, coriander, cumin, dill, fennel, parsley

The herbs and spices listed next also have anti-cancer actions: onions, flax, turmeric, mints, rosemary, thyme, oregano, sage, basil, tarragon

Recommendations: Increase the use of all these herbs and spices daily in your cooking for both flavor enhancement and their phytochemical content to maximize potential cancer protective benefits. Some new information concerning garlic has shown that cutting or smashing whole garlic bulbs 10 minutes before heating them helps to preserve the bulb's anti-cancer properties.

✒ DINING OUT:
HOW TO MAINTAIN
AN ANTI-CANCER DIET

Wherever I speak, the most frequently asked question I receive is, "How do you eat out and still maintain your healthful diet?" That is an excellent question and represents a common problem. Surveys have demonstrated that almost 50 percent of our food dollars are spent in restaurants (or for take-out food). In addition, we are eating out an average of three to four times each week.

Perhaps the hardest part of modifying your diet to reduce your cancer risk is deciding what to eat while away from home. How closely you maintain your diet while eating out is up to you, and it may depend on how often you eat out (or take-out). If you eat several meals away from home each week, or if you travel often, it may be especially important to choose wisely. Two important goals to keep in mind are minimizing your fat intake (for information on which types of fats are most harmful or beneficial, see pages 25 to 26) and emphasizing foods from plant sources (fruits, vegetables, nuts, grains and legumes) in your meals.

Additionally, remember to keep serving sizes in line when eating out. (See page 28 regarding what counts as a serving size.) Restaurants have dramatically increased portion sizes in recent years, which has been one factor contributing to America's expanding waist size, thereby increasing cancer risk.

Choose:	Limit:
Vegetables	Meats, poultry
Garden salad	Full-fat dairy products
Mixed greens	Cream sauce
Fruit	Cheese sauce
Whole grains, starches	Hollandaise
Beans, lentils	Alfredo
Nuts, seeds	Béarnaise
Seafood (fresh or water pack)	Au gratin
Low-fat dairy	Parmigiana
Egg whites/substitutes	Croquettes
Herbs and spices	Fritters
Marinara	Filo
Tomato sauce or base	Crispy, flaky
Light wine sauce	Batter-dipped, breaded
Steamed	Deep-fried
Baked, broiled	Tempura
Grilled	Escalloped
Poached	Newburg
Roasted	Scampi
Stewed	Blackened, charbroiled
Sautéed	Smoked
Stir-fried	Lard
Olive or canola oil (< 1 tsp.)	Vegetable oil
Condiments:	*Condiments:*
Salsa	Butter, margarine
Low-fat mayo or salad dressing	Full-fat mayo or salad dressing
Vinegar	Full-fat sour cream
Lemon juice	Full-fat cream cheese
Soy sauce	"Special sauce"
Cocktail sauce	Tartar sauce
Ketchup	Guacamole (small amounts OK)
Barbecue/steak sauce	
Mustard	
Pickle relish	
Pepper	
Jam/syrup/honey	

Helpful Tips

♦ Think "Ethnic": Ethnic restaurants are more likely to offer a wide variety of plant-based menu items. Chinese, Mexican, and Italian are the most common ethnic choices in the U.S., but many larger cities also offer Indian, Middle Eastern, Japanese, Thai, Korean, or Ethiopian fare. Challenge yourself to try new foods!

♦ Have a Plan: To select a restaurant, look in the Yellow Pages of the phone book or ask friends or family members (or, if you are traveling, a hotel manager or desk clerk) for suggestions. If you are trying a new restaurant, call ahead to ask what low-fat or vegetarian choices they offer or would be willing to prepare. You can also pick up a copy of their menu, ask them to fax it to you, or simply read over the menu before being seated. Frequent travelers may want to order a copy of *Vegetarian Journal's Guide to Natural Foods Restaurants in the US and Canada* (see references).

♦ Make the Best of it: If you are traveling and have limited restaurant choices (for example, at a rest stop on the highway), try to find a chain or fast food restaurant that you know offers menu items which fit into your healthy diet. The Vegetarian Resource Group has some very helpful guides for anyone who is trying to eat vegetarian at fast food or chain restaurants (see references).

♦ Be Creative: Even if there are no entrées on the menu that fit into your diet, you may be able to create a healthy meal out of several side dishes, appetizers, or soup and salad. Many salad bars offer a variety of healthy items. You may want to see what is available at the salad bar before you order.

♦ Share/Save the Sinful: If you can't resist ordering an entrée or a dessert that does not fit into your healthy diet, see if someone will share it with you. Then order a healthy entrée and/or salad or soup to go with it. If you will be dining alone, ask for a doggie bag (or box) and save the rest for later.

♦ Bring Your Own: If you're going someplace where you're not sure what you'll find to eat, or if you're headed to a junk food haven, bring your own healthy meals or snacks in your briefcase, purse, or backpack (see "Travel Tips" for suggestions for what to bring). Store food in a cooler for longer outings or vacations. If you'll be staying in a hotel, call ahead to ask if there will be a mini fridge in your room. This will give you more options for keeping your own food on hand.

♦ Just Ask: If you are unsure whether or not an item is vegetarian or if you would like to know how something is prepared, ask your server. He or she should either be able to tell you or find out for you. It may be harder to get information from fast food restaurants, although some, such as Subway and Wendy's, do provide nutritional information right in the store. If you still have questions, you can ask the manager for the phone number of the chain's corporate headquarters.

❧ **Make a Request:** Most any restaurant will respond to requests to modify an item, for example leaving the butter off your vegetables, putting your salad dressing on the side, or leaving the meat or dairy out of certain dishes. You may want to emphasize that these requests are for your health. At some of the more upscale restaurants, the chef may be able to prepare a special meal for you, such as a vegetable stir-fry or a tomato-based pasta dish with vegetables. If possible, you may want to call the restaurant ahead of time to make a special request, especially during busy times (*i.e.* Friday or Saturday night). If the restaurants you frequent have a limited selection of healthy items, encourage them to offer more choices.

Hidden Fat Traps and Vegetarian Concerns

❧ Refried beans often contain lard. Be sure to ask.

❧ Many soups, such as vegetable and bean soups, and rice dishes which appear to be vegetarian contain meat, meat stock, or animal fat.

❧ Some house salads are served with bacon bits, cheese, or egg. You should be able to order your salad without one or all of these items.

❧ Many sauces, including pasta and even pizza sauces, may contain meat, cheese, meat stocks, or animal fats. When in doubt, ask!

❧ Steamed vegetables and grilled fish often have butter added for flavor and moisture. Ask to have this omitted.

Salad Bar Tips

❧ Emphasize dark greens (romaine, spinach) vs. iceberg

❧ Load up on fruit (fresh if available)

❧ Top salads with a variety of veggies (shredded carrots, bell peppers, tomatoes, broccoli, cauliflower, cucumbers, mushrooms, green peas, sprouts, etc.)

❧ Add some garbanzo beans, kidney beans, and/or sunflower seeds for extra fiber and protein

---

❦ Skip the creamy, full-fat dressings and choose low-fat or fat-free dressing or a small amount of oil—preferably olive or canola—and vinegar. Or try substituting lemon juice or salsa with some pepper.

❦ *Suggestion:* Carry a very small container of olive oil in your purse, briefcase, or backpack to use with vinegar on your salad.

Avoid/Limit: creamy mixed salads such as potato salad, pasta salads, and coleslaw

Beverage Suggestions

❦ Water or mineral water with a slice of fruit

❦ Fruit/vegetable juices

❦ Iced tea

❦ Hot tea (green, herbal, black)

❦ Milk (low-fat or skim)

❦ Soy milk (from home)

❦ *Suggestion:* If you drink coffee, add soymilk, skim or low-fat milk instead of cream, or drink it black.

Meal Suggestions for a Low-Fat, Plant-Based Diet

❦ *Asian*

Examples are Chinese, Korean, Japanese, Thai, Vietnamese and Mongolian, which vary significantly. There should be many choices that emphasize vegetables and/or tofu. Request minimal oil or steamed for all dishes.

• Miso soup
• Sushi (can be ordered vegetarian),
• Steamed vegetable spring rolls
• Steamed rice (brown if available) or pasta
• Mu Shu with vegetables or seafood
• Spicy tofu, vegetables, or seafood
• Steamed vegetable dumplings (pot stickers)
• California rolls
• Cabbage or mixed green salads (with minimal or no oil)
• Teriyaki fish with vegetables
• Broth-based soups with vegetables, seaweed, seafood, rice or noodles

- Brown, Szechuan, Hunan, black bean or garlic sauce
- Stir-fried or steamed vegetables and bean curd (tofu) or seafood
- Fresh fruit
- Green or oolong tea

Avoid/Limit: Fried egg rolls, wontons, fried rice and noodles, dishes which emphasize meat—especially duck, beef, or pork, egg foo young, deep fried or breaded and fried dishes, tempura, dishes with coconut milk, teas made with cream or whole milk.

ᴥ *Italian*

- Bread with a touch of olive oil
- Fresh fruit
- Raw vegetables
- Steamed or roasted vegetables
- Bean salads
- Seafood cacciatore
- Green salad with olive oil and vinegar or low-fat dressing on the side
- Lentil or minestrone soup (may contain meat/meat stock)
- Pasta e fagioli (pasta and beans, note: may not be vegetarian)
- Pasta with marinara, tomato, or wine sauce or small amounts of pesto sauce
- Pasta primavera (with tomato or wine—not cream—base)
- Steamed or baked (not fried) eggplant or zucchini with tomato sauce

Avoid/Limit: Buttered garlic bread, meatballs, Italian sausage, veal dishes, pasta stuffed with meats or cheeses, cream sauces such as Alfredo or carbonara, sauces with meat or cheese, parmigiana or breaded and fried meats or vegetables.

ᴥ *Mexican*

- Green salad
- Steamed vegetables
- Fresh fruit
- Bean burrito
- Veggie or seafood fajita
- Bean taco or tostada
- Spanish rice
- Black beans (may come as a side dish)
- Gazpacho—request no sour cream or have it on the side
- Bean, vegetable, or seafood enchilada (with tomato-based—not cheese—sauce)
- Refried beans (make sure they're not cooked in lard or fat)

- Huevos rancheros (small portion—*i.e.* one egg—without cheese)
- Peppers—all varieties
- Toppings: salsa, salsa verde, picante sauce, lettuce, tomato, peppers, onions, small amounts of guacamole

Avoid/Limit: Fried tortilla chips, taco salads, beef tacos, deep-fried tacos or tortillas (chimichangas), chili con carne, sausage, fried chile rellenos, full-fat cheeses and cheese sauces, full-fat sour cream, deep fried ice cream.

🍎 Indian—Nepalese food is similar.

There should be many choices which emphasize vegetables, legumes, and herbs

- Vegetable raita salads (usually made with cucumbers and yogurt)
- Mixed vegetable salads
- Chapati and naan bread (not fried)
- Dahl (lentil) dishes
- Tomato-based dishes
- Basmati rice with vegetables
- Saffron rice
- Vegetable biryani
- Vegetable curries
- Aloo ghobi
- Steamed vegetable dumplings
- Masala sauce
- Chutneys (mango, onion, or mint)
- Fresh fruit
- Chai made with skim or soy milk

Avoid/Limit: Samosas, pakoras, dishes which emphasize meat—especially beef or lamb, heavy cream sauces, dishes cooked with butter or ghee, paneer (Indian cheese), fried breads, lassi (sweet yogurt drink), chai made with cream or whole milk.

🍎 Middle Eastern

Should offer plenty of vegetable- and lentil-based entrees

- Greek salad (without feta, or ask for a small amount of feta on the side)
- Grape leaves (stuffed with rice, tomato and onion. Note: some may have meat)
- Lentil or black bean soup

- Fattoush salad
- Tomato and cucumber salads
- Tabouli
- Rice
- Pita bread (whole wheat if available)
- Baba ghanouj
- Hummus
- Mujadara
- Baked (not fried) falafel
- Vegetable moussaka
- Vegetable boreks
- Dried fruit

Avoid/Limit: Meat dishes, high-fat (filo) spinach pies, deep-fried falafel, baklava.

🍎 American, European, or Bar and Grill

- Garden or side salad—ask for low-fat dressing on the side or oil and vinegar
- Steamed vegetables (some are prepared with butter or creamy sauces)
- Soups: Broth/tomato based, vegetable, lentil or bean (may not be vegetarian)
- Veggie sandwich or roll-up (some have cheese or mayo)
- Egg white or egg substitute omelet—no cheese, lots of veggies
- Pizza with no cheese or "half the cheese" and veggies (see "Pizza Place" suggestions)
- Baked potato—try salsa as a topping instead of sour cream and butter
- Pasta with marinara sauce
- Stir-fried vegetables with rice or pasta
- Grilled, broiled or poached salmon or tuna
- Veggie burger
- Rice pilaf (may not be vegetarian)
- Raw vegetables
- Fruit
- Low- or non-fat yogurt or sorbet

Avoid/Limit: Large portions of meat, especially red meats—such as hamburgers, sausages or ham, full-fat cheeses and cheese sauces, cream sauces, most fried foods (especially deep-fried or breaded and fried), and high-fat condiments (see "General Guidelines").

❝ Pizza Places/Sub Shops

- Garden or side salad (order without cheese or meat)
- Greek salad (without feta cheese or dressing, or a small amounts on the side)
- Pizza: Get hand-tossed or thin crust, not deep-dish or pan-fried
- Get a cheeseless pizza, or ask for less cheese or "half the cheese"
- Add lots of veggies, such as broccoli, green peppers, tomatoes, spinach, onions, olives, mushrooms, and artichoke hearts. Also try pineapple!
- Pasta with marinara sauce (may not be vegetarian)
- Vegetarian sub with no cheese or "half the cheese," light mayo or dressing (or mustard) and lots of veggies
- Veggie "pizza" sub with no cheese or "half the cheese" and lots of veggies
- Tuna sub made with low-fat mayo or dressing, and lots of veggies
- Suggestion: If you want meat on your sub, stick with a lower-fat choice such as turkey or chicken breast, and ask for half the standard amount of meat (and cheese) and extra veggies.

Avoid/Limit: Buttery/cheesy bread sticks, buttered garlic bread, French fries (especially chili cheese fries), chef salads, potato/snack chips, meat toppings on pizza, meat subs—especially Italian, ham, salami, meatball, and steak subs, ribs, chicken wings, pasta dishes with meats/cheeses, most desserts.

❝ Delis/Bagel Shops

- Garden or side salad
- Vegetarian Grape leaves
- Bean or lentil salads
- Tabouli
- Greek salad (without feta cheese, or a small amount of feta on the side)
- Low-fat or fat-free salad dressing or small amount of oil with vinegar
- Pasta, potato, rice, or tofu salads made with low-fat dressings
- Cooked seasoned vegetables (not in creamy or oily sauces)
- Soups: Broth- or tomato-based vegetable, lentil or bean (may not be vegetarian)
- Sandwiches:
  Bread, bagel, pita or roll (wheat or whole grain if available)
  Vegetarian (with no cheese or "half the cheese")
  Hummus
  Tuna made with low-fat mayo or dressing
  Lots of veggies (lettuce, tomatoes, peppers, onions, olives, etc.)
  Low-fat mayo or dressing, mustard

- Spaghetti with marinara sauce
- Hot baked potatoes (plain)
- Soft pretzel with mustard
- Low-fat yogurt
- Low-fat frozen yogurt with fresh fruit
- ***Suggestion:*** If you want meat on your sandwich, stick with a lower-fat choice such as turkey or chicken breast, and ask for half the standard amount of meat (and cheese) and extra veggies.

Notes:

At grocery stores these items may be found behind the deli counter or prepackaged in cases near the deli. Some items may be located elsewhere in the store, such as near the produce section.

Be sure to check dates on prepackaged items before buying them. Also, feel free to ask the deli server for suggestions (what is fresh, what they recommend, etc.) before you order.

For other healthy grocery items, check for a "health food" section. Soy products, such as soymilk and baked tofu, and organic dairy products are now available in many "mainstream" grocery stores.

Many grocery store delis are now featuring take-out meals. Be sure to check ingredient labels, as many of these items are not low fat. For example, potatoes may be mashed with whole milk and butter, or twice baked with cheese and sour cream.

Avoid/Limit: Full-fat creamy potato or pasta salads and coleslaws, chef salads, potato/snack chips, sandwiches with meat—especially bacon, salami, pastrami, ham and cheese, or corned beef, and most desserts and baked goods, including brownies, cheesecake, cookies, croissants, and regular (full-fat) muffins.

❦ *Breakfast/Bakeries*

Breakfast bars may have a variety of cold cererals and fresh fruit

- Oatmeal (or other whole-grain hot cereals)—with low/non-fat milk, or soy milk (bring from home)
- Cold cereals—whole grain, such as Raisin Bran®, All Bran®, Wheaties®, or Cheerios®
- Low-fat fruit or bran muffin
- Fresh fruit and fruit juices
- Dry wheat toast with or without jam—ask for no butter
- Bagel or English muffin with or without jam—ask for no butter

- Pancakes or waffles without butter (may contain eggs and dairy)—with fruit
- Egg white or egg substitute omelets—ask for no cheese, lots of veggies
- Roasted or boiled potatoes (ask if there is added fat)
- Low-fat yogurt

Avoid/Limit: Bacon, ham, sausage, large omelets with meats/cheeses, quiches, croissants, regular (full-fat) muffins, deep-fried French toast, granola (unless it's low-fat), whole milk, cream, hash browns, fried potatoes.

❖ Fast Food

- Garden or side salad (without cheese) with fat-free or low-fat dressing (Note: Many are mainly iceberg lettuce, which is low in nutrients and cancer-fighting phytochemicals)
- Baked potato (no cheese sauce, or cheese sauce on the side) with broccoli and/or salsa
- Bean burrito or taco—ask for beans instead of beef, no cheese, and extra veggies
- Low-fat submarine sandwiches (see "Sub Shop" suggestions above)
- Low-fat bagel sandwiches (see "Bagel Shop" suggestions above)
- Veggie pita—no added sauce, or low-fat sauce on the side
- Burgerless burger (bun, lettuce, onions, extra tomatoes, ketchup and mustard, with or without cheese and mayo or special sauce)
- Grilled or broiled chicken sandwich with low-fat sauce or sauce on the side
- Pasta bar—choose tomato-based sauces, avoid meat/cheese/cream sauces
- Salad bar—See "Salad Bar Tips" on pages 49-50. Avoid chef salads, taco salads, and regular (full-fat) salad dressings

- Fast Food Breakfast Options:
  Low-fat bran muffin
  Cereal (such as Cheerios®) with low-fat milk (or soy milk from home)
  English muffin with or without jam—ask for no butter
  Pancakes with syrup (may contain eggs and dairy)—ask for no butter
  Low-fat yogurt
  Orange or other fruit juice

Avoid/Limit: Burgers—especially double or quarter-pound burgers, deep-fried chicken or fish sandwiches, chicken nuggets, mayo, cheese, cheese sauce, special sauce, sour cream, French fries, snack chips, whole milk, milkshakes made with whole milk or oil, most (especially deep-fried) desserts, breakfast pastries, egg/meat biscuits, super size or deluxe meals.

✎ Gas Stations/Convenience Stores

Although some convenience stores may have prepackaged sandwiches, they usually don't have many healthy choices for meals. If you do stop at a convenience store for snacks, here are some of the better choices:

- Mixed nuts, cashews, peanuts, sunflower seeds or pumpkin seeds (dry roasted if available)
- Fig bars (fat-free if available)
- Dried fruit
- Low-fat, whole grain crackers
- Low-fat "breakfast" or granola bars
- Pretzels
- Whole grain cereals
- Fruit/vegetable juices

Sample Menus

The following menus were designed to provide suggestions for maintaining a low-fat, plant-based diet for those times when your only meal choices may be chain or fast food restaurants. They represent some of the best choices available from a limited selection of healthy menu items. (Special Note: Some of the menu items used as examples may not be available.)

Day 1: Chain Restaurants:

Breakfast: Big Boy's
Bowl of oatmeal—skim milk on side (or bring your own soymilk)
Fresh strawberries
Wheat toast (no butter) with jam
Grapefruit juice

Lunch: Olive Garden
Capellini Pomodoro (angel hair pasta with tomatoes and Romano
    cheese)
Minestrone soup
Plain breadstick (ask for no butter)
Ice water

Dinner: Applebee's
Low-Fat Veggie Quesadilla (comes with non-fat cheese and sour
    cream)
Steamed broccoli and carrots (special request)
Hot or iced tea

Snacks: from home or grocery

One peeled orange
Two T. roasted soy nuts or soy nut butter
10 whole grain crackers
8 oz. soymilk box
Plenty of fresh water

Nutritional Value:

Provides approximately four servings of fruits, five servings of vegetables, 10 servings of grains (including two whole grains), and two to three servings of soy. Provides approximately 2,000 calories, 90 grams of protein, 40 grams of fat, 30 grams of fiber, and 18 percent of calories from fat.

Note: Items may be added or deleted to meet higher or lower calorie needs.

Day 2: Fast Food Restaurants:

Breakfast: McDonald's
Lowfat Apple Bran Muffin
Cheerios® with 1 percent milk (or bring your own soy milk)
Large orange juice

Lunch: Wendy's
Garden Veggie Pita, no added dressing
Fruit juice

Dinner: Subway
Veggie Delite™ 12" Sub—without cheese
Iced or hot tea or water

Snacks-from home or grocery
1/2 c. carrot sticks or baby carrots
1 apple
8 oz. soy drink box
2 T. roasted soy nuts
Plenty of fresh water

Nutritional Value:

Provides approximately four servings of fruits, four to five servings of vegetables, 13 servings of grains (10 whole grains), and two to three servings of soy. Provides approximately 1,850 calories, 60 grams of protein, 30 grams of fat, 25 grams of fiber, and 15 percent of calories from fat.

Travel Tips—
Ideas for Eating on the Road or Bringing Your Own Food

- Whole grain bread or bagels (for sandwiches)
- Instant or prepared hummus, for sandwiches or a veggie dip (should be kept cold once prepared)
- Soy nut butter, to spread on sandwiches, crackers, or fruit
- Small cans of beans with pop-up lids
- Small cans of water-pack tuna with pop-up lids
- Fresh veggies such as baby carrots, carrot sticks or pepper slices
- Fresh fruits, such as bananas, apples, pears, oranges, peaches, nectarines or plums
- Small cans of fruit (preferably in fruit juice or "lite" syrup) with pop-up lids
- Fresh fruit salad (store in airtight container)
- Dried fruits, such as raisins, figs, or apricots
- Cups of low-fat or soy yogurt (keep cold)
- Small boxes of whole grain cold cereals
- Nutlettes Plus® cereal—makes its own soy milk (see references for order info.)
- Instant cups of soup
- Instant cups of hot whole grain cereal
- Low-fat, whole-grain muffins or quickbreads—such as pumpkin or banana (homemade)
- Popcorn—preferably air-popped or popped in olive or canola oil
- Low-fat, whole grain crackers or pretzels
- Roasted soy nuts
- Dry-roasted nuts or seeds
- Soy drink boxes
- Fruit/vegetable juices
- Plenty of fresh water
- Iced tea and/or tea bags to make hot tea
- Small container of olive oil for salad dressing and/or bread in restaurants that only have vegetable oil

You may want to stop at grocery stores along the way to pick up extra snacks, or healthy meals from the deli or salad bar. Farmers' markets or roadside stands are also good places to stock up on fresh fruits and veggies. Bring whatever you will need for preparation or consumption of your meals (*i.e.* cutting knife, utensils, napkins, plates or bowls, cups or mugs, storage containers).

Airlines: Most airline flights no longer have meals available. If they do, the Vegetarian Resource Group (see references) recommends requesting a special meal when you make your reservation and then again 24 hours before your flight is scheduled to leave. Choices may include bland-soft, diabetic, Kosher, low fat, low sodium, low cholesterol, vegetarian with dairy, vegan (no eggs or dairy), or fruit plate.

Some international flights also offer special ethnic meals, which may include additional vegetarian options. The best choices for a low-fat, plant-based meal will most likely be vegan, fruit plate, or vegetarian ethnic options. Another option is to bring your own meal or snacks. It's a good idea to do this anyway, to ensure that you'll have something to eat in case, for whatever reason, you don't get your meal. Also, be sure to stay well hydrated; take advantage of the beverage service or bring your own water or other non-caffeinated beverages, such as fruit or vegetable juices.

Special Note: If you will be crossing international borders, be sure to check on regulations for bringing food into the country.

Conclusion

Once you begin to learn what choices are available at various restaurants, and what the healthiest options are, the task of maintaining your anti-cancer diet while eating out should become easier. You may even find that it is fun to experiment with new foods at ethnic restaurants! Although it is certainly a challenge to find healthy foods while eating out, it doesn't have to be a chore. Check out some of the resources listed on pages 113 to 114 for further suggestions. Happy (and healthy) dining!

This chapter, "Dining Out: How to Maintain Your Anti-Cancer Diet", was written in 1998 by Sara Post Chatfield, MPH, RD, as part of her graduate studies at The University of Michigan under the supervision of Diana Dyer, MS, RD.

MY "DECISION TREE" FOR EVALUATING AND IMPLEMENTING ANY ALTERNATIVE THERAPY

When I have worked at hospitals in the past, patients would occasionally bring in a large number of various dietary supplements that they wished to continue taking while hospitalized. At that time, this was my only exposure and source of information about the entire world of alternative medicine and to step into that world myself made me more than a little uneasy. However, since I had decided to make significant changes to my diet, I was now very curious about what else was out there that offered promise to help reduce my risk for cancer recurrence.

My initial goal was to enhance my immune system to its maximum potential in order to help reduce my chances for cancer returning. During the 10+ years between my two breast cancers, my white blood cell counts never reached the normal range of 4,000 to 10,000. Mine were always 2,000 to 2,500 and occasionally even lower. The explanation given to me was these low counts were to be expected due to the amount of damage my bone marrow had sustained from both the radiation treatments that cured me of my childhood cancer and the chemotherapy that helped cure me of my first breast cancer. As a clinical scientist, I had always accepted that explanation as a reasonable consequence of past successes. However, after my third cancer, the patient part of my brain took over, and I no longer felt I could afford to accept that limitation as a given. I was ready to try multiple means to augment my immune system—direct changes by altering my diet and introducing some herbs and vitamins, and indirect changes by some mind-body-spirit connection techniques.

I read extensively for the first year while I was making the changes in my diet. It would have been too overwhelming for me to change everything at once. Besides, I wanted to try to sort out what might offer some real hope.

As I read, I developed goals I wanted to achieve along with the following thought process for myself to evaluate which strategies might be helpful for me. You may also think of other important questions to ask. In addition, these questions could also be applied to conventional therapies:

- Is there scientific evidence that this therapy will reduce/eliminate breast tumors of my type and stage (or your type of cancer) in humans? What is the strength of the evidence? How does it work?

- Is there any evidence that this therapy may be potentially harmful for me?

- Is there evidence that this supplement or technique is harmless, or at the very best may increase my quality of life?

- Instead of supplementation, is there a way to obtain the same (or better) result from food sources?

- How much money was I able and willing to spend not reimbursed by medical insurance?

- Does this therapy feel right in my heart/gut? Does this therapy speak to me? This question is important. It has allowed me to proceed with a therapy before having all the other questions answered to the satisfaction of my "left brain."

- Who should I choose as a practitioner/therapist/healer? What are their qualifications and my comfort level with them?

- Time considerations—"natural healing" takes time and effort—was I willing to invest that time and work for healing?

- Discuss this therapy with your oncologist or primary care physician. They may have some valid concerns regarding your particular medical condition. Become a full and equal partner on your medical team.

I cannot emphasize enough the importance of discussing all available therapeutic options, both conventional and complementary, with your physicians. Even if your physician never asks if you are interested and/or are already incorporating some complementary strategies into your cancer action plan, it is your responsibility to inform him/her. Speaking for myself, that takes courage! I found the courage because I have the conviction that these additional therapies are as important to my healing as the conventional therapies, and I wanted my physician to know that.

♋ DIETARY SUPPLEMENTS

The following list is my current individual regimen for enhancing my body's anti-oxidant and immune systems. Does every cancer patient need these supplements or perhaps different ones or amounts? I don't know the full answer to that, and I don't believe anyone else does either. However, it now seemed apparent to me that a person like myself, with a tendency for developing cancer, needed something more than what I was getting from my previously healthy diet alone if I stood a chance to keep cancer from returning again. (I want to emphasize though that I think of these supplements as just that—supplements to help my ultra-healthy diet for optimal health, not magic bullets expected to compensate for an unhealthy diet and lifestyle.)

There is currently much controversy surrounding the pros and cons of taking anti-oxidants while also receiving chemotherapy or radiation. It is not fully understood at this time if large doses of antioxidants may protect cancer cells from the intended effects from chemo or radiation therapy, act as pro-oxidants causing more damage than protection of our healthy cells, or even act to enhance the effects of radiation or chemotherapy. It is highly likely to be very individualistic depending on tumor type and staging, drug mechanism of action, and many different individual biochemical characteristics. Research needs to be carried out evaluating combinations of anti-oxidants, not just individual anti-oxidants, and I hope much more research is done to determine the optimal supplementation beneficial for various cancers and each type of therapy.

I did not take any supplements at all while I was on chemotherapy. I began taking supplements only after my chemotherapy was finished. If you have a decreased nutritional intake during your cancer therapy, taking a one-a-day type of supplement providing 100 percent of the RDAs of vitamins and minerals is appropriate. Additionally, ask to see the dietitian at your cancer center for guidance about up-to-date research on this topic.

- ♥ Multi-vitamin and mineral supplement with approximately 100 percent RDA of everything—a brand with a lower amount of iron (10 milligrams or less per tablet)

- ♥ Vitamin C—250 milligrams once per day

- ♥ Vitamin E—200 IU—one time per day—take with a meal or snack containing some fat to maximize absorption. Check expiration date of bottle. I use a natural (d-alpha) Vitamin E containing mixed tocopherols.

- Calcium—600 to 1200 milligrams per day—for my osteoporosis. I use calcium citrate with additional vitamin D.

- Vitamin D3 (cholecalciferol)—1000 to 2000 IU per day

- Co-enzyme Q10—100 milligrams per day. An antioxidant. Optimal dosing to help prevent recurrence is not known yet. I based my dosage on what I am willing to spend per month.

Although I am now officially a "pill popper," I still believe the overall health benefits I am receiving from my nine+ servings of fruits and vegetables and one to three servings of soy foods each day are even more important than the benefits of these supplements. If I were forced to choose only one approach, I would put my money on maximizing my diet for the largest potential benefit.

HOW TO CHOOSE A BRAND OF VITAMIN OR HERB

The choices available in the health food or grocery store are overwhelming. Here are some general guidelines to help you choose a quality product.

Vitamins and Minerals:

1. Choose a supplement with the USP notation on the label. Having this on the label means the company is legally responsible to the FDA for meeting dissolution standards, which means the product has been tested to ensure it will actually disintegrate in your body. Additionally, this product has been tested to determine that the amounts indicated on the label are actually in the supplement and have met purity standards. Only the term USP guarantees that these important standards have been met.

2. The USP dissolution standard has not been tested with sustained or timed release products.

3. Check the expiration date. I have seen stores selling vitamins in a two-for-one sale that were very close to the expiration date.

4. Take your vitamin or mineral supplement with food. That is especially important with fat-soluble vitamins that need to be in the presence of fat to be absorbed.

(Source: *Tufts University Health and Nutrition Letter*, November 1997)

Herbs and other Dietary Supplements:

Currently, there are no regulations in effect that assure consumers of either the quantity or quality of herbs or other dietary supplements being purchased. *Consumer's Report* has published their investigative research showing widely varying contents (quantity and purity) of various dietary supplements bought from retail stores. Standardization of a product is optional at this time, and indeed, there are widely differing (and contentious) views among herbalists about the pros and cons of standardizing herbs for only one active constituent.

A company called ConsumerLab.com does independent testing of dietary supplements for accuracy of contents. In other words, is what's listed on the label what is actually in those capsules? Common products of herbal supplements, vitamin products, and other dietary supplements are bought from retailers and tested. Results from the testing, including brand names for products that had accurate labeling, are posted on the company's web site at www.consumerlab.com. New testing is being done regularly, so this is a very valuable web site to keep checking.

A trade organization called the National Nutritional Foods Association has recently developed its own guidelines called Good Manufacturing Practices (GMP). NNFA's GMP program requires third-party inspections of manufacturing facilities to determine whether NNFA-specified standards are being met. These standards include specifications for testing of raw and finished materials, staff training, cleanliness, equipment maintenance and record keeping. All member companies of NNFA that manufacture dietary supplements will be required to meet these guidelines and pass these inspections at which point they will be eligible to display a GMP seal on the labels of their products. It is important to remember that passing this inspection process is not a stamp of approval on the efficacy of this product (*i.e.*, has it been proven to be beneficial in particular clinical situations?) but simply on the manufacturing of the product.

Most recently, NSF International has developed a Dietary Supplements Certification Program, a voluntary program created with input by all interested parties (from growers through consumers) that will provide very thorough testing of dietary supplements. This newest certification process is the most rigorous one developed to date. Look for dietary supplements that have a NSF logo on the front. NSF's Web site will list the products as they become certified (www.nsf.org).

I suggest calling the company that makes the dietary supplements you purchase to ask how their products are certified. This is an important first step. There is still a lot of reading you must do to determine if a product will be helpful to you (fits with your goals). However, a certification program like NSF's will help you feel more confidant that a product you purchase will actually contain what is stated on the label (both nothing more and nothing less).

Some additional advice is the importance of keeping a diary or log of all the supplements you are consuming, including brand name, dosage, frequency, along with recording any signs, symptoms, or changes they might notice that should be brought to the attention of their cancer team members. In addition, if you are starting a new complementary therapy such as acupuncture, meditation, yoga, guided imagery, etc., keep records of when you started that, too, along with any changes you observe. All of this information should be incorporated into your medical records because all of these strategies are contributing to your healing.

It is also advisable to introduce or change only one new herb, supplement, or therapy at a time. I recommend waiting three to four days at a minimum. That way the development of any adverse effects can be more easily traced to a particular change or addition, just like with a medication. If you do develop any unusual side effects or symptoms, stop your supplements and notify your physician(s) and any additional health care practitioner who is guiding you on choices of complementary therapies.

You may self-report any adverse reactions to drugs, herbs, and other dietary supplements to the FDA's Medwatch by calling 1-800-332-1088. In addition, the Web sites www.safetyalerts.com and www.consumerlab.com tell if a particular dietary supplement has been recalled.

ADDITIONAL INGREDIENTS IN MY HEALING RECIPE

Besides changing my diet and adding some supplements, I have also included multiple new ingredients into my life to fully heal from this latest cancer—healing physically, emotionally, mentally, and spiritually. Going through this for the third time now gave me reason to begin looking at everything in my life. I intuitively knew that I could not just jump back into my previous routines this time.

Recovering cancer patients should do a life review no matter what their age. In my case, I was 45 years old and really primed for a monumental mid-life evaluation. Everything was fair game—should I keep it, keep it as is or change it, should I pitch it, what was new that I should add? As I mentioned earlier, this process was even more difficult for me than completing chemotherapy. I don't say that to discourage you—only to give you fair notice. I wouldn't be writing about it if I didn't think the evaluation and searching process had value.

The following list includes the new additions to my life. Many of them are major lifestyle changes, such as daily meditation and exercise. These take time and a commitment to making the time to do them. Every component listed here is very meaningful and has helped me heal on multiple levels. Your list may look very different from mine, as there is more than one road to healing. I've included a lengthy list of the multiple ways different members of my support group are using to heal on page 75 to 76.

Don't ignore or suppress the need for full healing from your cancer experience at more than a physical level. I have chosen many of these activities because they address different levels of my healing needs. My needs were extensive because I had not really addressed them after my first two cancers. I had simply coped. Each of you is at a different place with your recovery. Hopefully, this book will give you some ideas and resources to begin (or continue) your own healing journey.

✦ Be outside daily experiencing God's beautiful natural world. Sometimes it is only to fill the bird feeders, but I get outside daily to offer my thanks for feeling the sun, wind, or rain on my face. Good research now shows the benefits of being in nature for cancer patients.

✦ Breast cancer support group—monthly. I didn't join one after my first breast cancer—I don't really know why. This time, after my second breast cancer, I initially went simply for information but eventually discovered what kept me going back was the love and support, the inspiration, that I received from everyone there. Now that I'm farther along with my recovery, I am in a position to offer both "information and inspiration" to new cancer survivors.

🍏 Cancer Survivors' Network—I joined the committee of a community-based group of cancer survivors that planned the activities for the local 1997 National Cancer Survivors' Day event and has also worked to identify and address the large unmet needs of cancer survivors in our community. This group is fun and stimulating. By developing friendships with men and women, old and young, all with different kinds of cancers, treatments, side effects, and inspirational stories to share, I have greatly broadened my horizons of understanding of both the difficulties and triumphs of being a cancer survivor.

Exercise

🍏 Walking briskly (combined with interspersed running) two to three miles per day five to seven times each week. As I mentioned previously, I was not faithful before, but now I'm outside exercising if it's above zero degrees with no ice. Otherwise, I will use an exercise bicycle or stair stepper inside. (Note—I now wear a warmer coat and use ice-grippers on my boots so I can be outside even on those very cold and icy days.) I also use strength-training exercises and do yoga three times per week to help improve my osteoporosis.

🍏 T'ai Chi—daily at home. I do these slow Chinese exercises using a video as a guide. I love the slow movement, the balancing, and slowing of my thoughts during the session. I always feel centered after completing this even though I would likely obtain even more benefit if I were in a group class receiving the energy of both my classmates and my teacher.

🍏 Qi gong (also called Chi Kung)—daily at home and once weekly in a group with a teacher. These are also Chinese exercises however Qi gong incorporates visualizations, and meditative breathing with the slow movements. Qi gong was developed thousands of years before T'ai Chi with the purpose of stimulating the body's self-healing potential. I have had some very profound and unexpected metaphysical experiences doing my Qi gong that I believe have been very instrumental with my healing. Interestingly, these happened even before I had learned that Qi gong is used in China in their cancer clinics.

🍏 Yoga—I am just starting to learn some beginning positions and movements, which are helping me build upper-body strength. Additionally, yoga has helped the aches still remaining in my upper arm after surgery finally disappear.

Homeopathic remedies as prescribed by my homeopathic physician.

I decided to make an appointment with a homeopathic physician after doing enough reading to accept that no homeopathic remedy prescribed was likely to be harmful. I don't fully understand how homeopathy works, but I believe that it might be helpful without being harmful or outrageously expensive. I also knew this physician was knowledgeable about many aspects of alternative medicine, and after talking with several people who went to him, I felt comfortable that he would be honest with me about "hope vs. hype." He also was forthright about discussing potential dangers various alternative approaches might have for me. Homeopathic remedies are prescribed on an individual basis, taking many factors into account. The ones prescribed for me for detoxification and osteoporosis support were all quite inexpensive. Although I did much of my own reading about herbs, he also has guided me in the selection of the few herbs I am taking.

Meditation—
Daily in A.M. for 30 to 45 Minutes (Ideal Would Be Two Times per Day).

I do "mindful meditation" every morning before my family gets up. I learned about meditation in an eight-session class entitled "The Magic of Healing." (See resource list for resources.) I have had several experiences while meditating that have positively impacted my healing. I apparently derive more benefit from meditating than I receive from the hour of sleep I give up, because I have found my body wakes up on its own ready to meditate no matter what time I went to bed. I believe that learning to meditate, and doing it faithfully, has been a very important change for me, as it is the time during which I listen to God.

Imagery

I have two sets of imagery that I do daily, which are my own visions of healing within my body. This takes 20 to 30 minutes daily following my meditation. I had read *Getting Well Again*, by Drs. Carl and Stephanie Simonton, when I underwent chemotherapy in 1984. As I went through chemotherapy the second time, I found myself automatically starting to use the techniques discussed in their book for developing images of my body healing itself.

Previously I had used their "Pac-Man" image for my white blood cells seeking and destroying the cancer cells in my body. However, in 1995, I needed to change the image to something more personal to me. Swans returning in the spring have long been a symbol to me of rebirth and renewal. This time around, I preferred to image a swan, taking

"Pac-Man's" place, finding cancer cells to eat and thus eliminate from my body. Later after I began meditating, I had a "vision" of flocks and flocks of swans entering my body to help with this process. In addition, now the swans were not just in my blood stream but were everywhere throughout my tissues looking for cancer cells and eliminating them. During this portion of my imagery, I visit with my swans, feed them special treats, and tell them how grateful I am for their assistance. Because there are so many swans now, I know that they will take care of me, and I don't have to worry if I miss a day of doing my visualizations.

My second set of visualizations focus on my bone marrow, the site of white blood cell production, so critical to the healthy functioning of the immune system. I visualize my bone marrow as a large beautiful English garden, filled with colorful flowers, herbs, birds, honeybees, and ponds. I am the gardener whose job it is to keep everything beautiful and healthy. I nurture the garden (my bone marrow) as I cultivate, weed, water, mulch, prune, plant, transplant, and also simply sit in the sun and enjoy its sights, smell, and sounds. It's one of my dream jobs, I love being there.

Hypnotherapy

I listen to a self-guided cassette tape, individualized for me, once or twice each week before I go to sleep at night. When I wake up the next morning, I am always astounded by the sense of energy that I feel. I met a local certified hypnotherapist who works extensively with cancer patients only after the *Detroit Free Press* article was published. I am now curious whether this therapy would have helped me have more energy during chemotherapy!

Feng Shui Consultation and Evaluation of My Home

Feng Shui is the ancient Chinese practice of assessing and altering various aspects of your physical surroundings (furniture placement, colors, aromas, shapes, etc.) in order to balance and maximize your internal energy or "Chi." This was a fun thing to do, and we are slowly making some changes in our home as a result of this consult. Some of the suggestions didn't sit well with me, but that's OK. It's important to listen to those inner feelings, too.

Shiatsu

Based on traditional Chinese medicine, shiatsu is an ancient form of hands-on therapy that enlists pressure point massage and stretching to balance the flow of Chi throughout the body. I am intuitively drawn to many facets of Chinese healing and have just started going to a shiatsu practitioner. I have experienced relief from some significant physical pains remaining in my arm following surgery, but even more interesting to me have been the flashes of new insight that have occurred while having this therapy done.

Prayer

I prayed before this latest cancer and chemotherapy but, just like with my exercising, I was not faithful about it. I now pray daily, in fact many times throughout the day. I pray everyday with thankfulness for my life along with prayers for guidance and strength that I might continue to do God's plan for me. It is also very meaningful to me to be able to pray for anyone who needs prayers, which includes my clients and even total strangers. I can tell you there are no words to express what it feels like to know that people all over the country are praying for you.

Reading

As strange as it may sound, I never read extensively about cancer or even the subject of cancer and nutrition during the 10+ years between my two breast cancers. I was immersed in a different subspecialty field of clinical nutrition that required substantial daily reading to remain current. However, in retrospect, I suspect I was in a state of denial about my cancer history.

I've now turned my voracious appetite for knowledge to strictly reading information regarding cancer, the nutrition and cancer connections, and the books that discuss the mind-body-spirit connection. I'm now also starting to mix in more inspirational books written by cancer survivors. I certainly haven't found nor had time to read all the best helpful books available. If you have a particular book to recommend, please let me know!

Gardening

There is a Chinese quotation that belongs in every garden, particularly a garden planted and tended by a cancer survivor:

"Life begins the day you plant a garden"

Why garden? Let me count the ways: the seed catalogs arriving, the dreaming, planning, seed ordering or plant purchasing, planting with your hands in the soil, weeding, watering, nurturing the soil and baby plants to fruition, harvesting, cooking, savoring the delicious eating, sharing the bounty, preserving, eating again during the winter, exercise, vitamin D, quality time with family and friends (even making new friends), the creation of something beautiful, a spiritual connection with our Mother Earth, and memories. All of those reasons, indeed any one of them, provide hope and purpose for the future, and they sound like the good life to me.

Years ago a friend who is also a cancer survivor 'confessed' to me that she stopped doing her daily meditation and yoga during the summer, hoping that the time she spent in her garden instead was 'good enough' to substitute for the benefits these practices provide. Her comment has stayed with me all these years, and in fact, was the starting point for my thoughts that gardening itself (not just being in or viewing nature), also provides a regular activity that engages and connects the body, mind, and spirit. Although only rarely listed or recommended as a complementary therapy for cancer patients, here is a classic example of "everything old is new again".

All of these thoughts inspired me to begin a new blog entitled "Cancer Victory Gardens™" at www.cancervictorygardens.com where I will be sharing my on-going thoughts about the benefits of gardening for cancer prevention, when under-going cancer treatments, and during the recovery time in order to help people "cultivate health through a garden's nourishment of both body and soul." Please feel free to share thoughts and experiences with your own Cancer Victory Garden™ at this blog.

I have shared with you all the various new ingredients that I added to my life in order to create my healing recipe. I kept many things in my life the same—my husband and sons, my friends, pets, fun, and vacations, which have also made major contributions to my overall successful recipe for healing. My recipe is only a guide. I have found there seem to be a few ingredients that are essential for me while others have some leeway. My days are never identical. Yet most everything gets done to some degree.

I am now more than 15 years past my latest cancer diagnosis in 1995. I feel wonderful everyday, better than I ever did in the 10+ years between my two breast cancers. I have tons of energy—I never nap—I am on the go until 11:00 each night. So far, there are no indications of a breast cancer recurrence or another new life-threatening cancer diagnosis. Perhaps something even more astonishing is the fact that some of my white blood cell counts have actually been within the normal range during my most recent recovery—something that was never accomplished during the 10+ years between my two breast cancers.

I have combined strategies from both medical worlds—conventional and complementary—to develop a truly integrated healing approach addressing all aspects of the mind-body-spirit connection. All the ingredients to my healing recipe have apparently worked together to create truly remarkable results. My oncologist is amazed and also impressed with the results I have been able to achieve. He even traveled to China to learn more about the traditional Chinese therapies, including herbs and Qi gong, used in China's cancer clinics in conjunction with the best of the conventional Western treatments. His hope is to learn how to combine the best of these therapies so that all cancer patients might benefit from this integrated approach to healing in the future.

🦢 TECHNIQUES AND TOOLS USED BY MY BREAST CANCER SUPPORT GROUP MEMBERS TO BOTH COPE AND HEAL

- Al Anon
- Any craft/art with tactile sense
- Art therapy
- Astragalus
- Ayruvedic medicine
- Belief that healing occurs at many levels and does not need to equate to a cure.
- Believe in your choices
- Birdwatching
- Cancer retreats
- Co-enzyme Q10, Pycnogenol, Aloe vera with Vitamin E
- Diet changes
- Echinacea
- Essiac tea
- Exercise
- Family
- Feng Shui
- Friends
- Fun!
- Gardening
- Guided imagery
- Guided imagery of cancer destruction, healing, and wellness and wholeness
- Healing music during surgery
- Homeopathy
- Humor
- Hydrazine sulfate
- Journaling
- Listening to yourself
- Macrobiotic diet
- Massage
- Meditation
- Music

- Organizing family photos
- Poetry writing
- Positive thinking
- Prayer
- Qi gong
- Reading for information and inspiration
- Reframing attitudes—victorious in cancer, not merely a survivor
- Relaxation
- Ritual of birthday celebrations
- Support groups
- Susan Wolf Sternberg's support groups and book, *A Year of Miracles*
- Tai Chi
- Taking one-step at a time
- Talking
- Therapeutic touch
- Yoga

This list shows a sample of the wide range of therapies that have been used to complement conventional treatments for cancer in order to help the whole person recover fully, to continue the journey of life in a meaningful and productive manner. (Inclusion of a therapy on this list is not intended as an endorsement by the author or publisher.)

🦢 FACTS, FIGURES, AND THOUGHTS

There are approximately 1,500 deaths from cancer daily in the U.S. (approximately one death each minute, or the same as the Titanic sinking every day!). However, I prefer to concentrate and visualize myself in the group of cancer survivors, of which there are now more than 12 million in the U.S. today, up from six million in 1990. Approximately six million of these survivors are now at least five years past their diagnosis. You are not alone, but instead are a member of quite a large club!

I would like to share the following quotations with you. They have been very meaningful to me as I have recovered from my latest cancer.

🍏 "Survivorship, quite simply, begins when you are told you have cancer and continues for the rest of your life." Fitzhugh Mullan, M.D. (cancer survivor and founder of the National Coalition of Cancer Survivorship)

🍏 "Cancer survivorship is dynamic as opposed to static; it is not just about long-term survival. It goes beyond the disease and the response—or lack of response—to treatment. Rather survivorship permeates every aspect of your life after diagnosis." Susan Leigh, RN, BSN (survivor of three different cancers)

🍏 "Successful survivorship does not need to equate to 'cure'. Healing is possible even when a cure is not." Michael Lerner, Ph.D. (founder of Commonweal, a cancer retreat center in California, and author, *Choices in Healing*)

🍏 "It is necessary to hope...for hope itself is happiness." Samuel Johnson

🍏 "Hope is the last to die." Russian Proverb

CHARACTERISTICS AND SKILLS OF SURVIVORS

I have been amazed to discover such an instant and deep bond with all of the cancer survivors who have called me, a total stranger, in response to the newspaper articles written about my life. As I talked to you and also thought about all the people I've known who have had cancer, I compiled a list of characteristics and skills that you all have demonstrated. I believe they are essential in order to maximize our chances of long-term survival, a sense of well being, and true healing. Not everyone has perfected all of these characteristics and skills (myself included), but they are worth working on.

Characteristics of Cancer Survivors:

- Communicator
- Desire and have the ability to move forward in life
- Desire to evolve beyond "just surviving" to "thriving"
- Flexible
- Forgiving
- Hopeful
- Information seeker
- Living life both joyfully and creatively
- Negotiator
- Out-spoken
- Persistent
- Pro-active
- Problem solver
- Resilient
- Resourceful
- Self advocate, indeed a full partner, in your medical care
- Self-reliant
- Sense of humor

I have also observed in some of you, and personally experienced myself, both denial and anger with our cancer diagnoses and all the resultant problems that must now be addressed. My own personal belief is that both of these reactions are appropriate and should not be suppressed. They are both very effective early coping tools and can serve a person well for a time. However, I believe for true healing to occur, a person must not get stuck in either of these two modes but must work to move beyond them in order to truly heal at all levels, physically, emotionally, mentally, and spiritually.

🦢 CLOSING THOUGHTS

This book, like my life, is a "work in progress" as I continue to fine-tune my own cancer recovery plan. There are undoubtedly many other helpful resources and therapies that also could have been included on this list. If you have read a book or tried a strategy that I have not mentioned that has been particularly helpful to you for your cancer recovery, please let me know. In addition, future and on-going research in nutrition, oncology, and alternative and complementary therapies will give us new information to incorporate into future cancer prevention, treatment, and recovery strategies.

I now understand there is no one absolute map for healing from cancer. Because each person is unique, every healing journey will be unique. I believe the seeking, the journey process itself, is as important to the ultimate healing of the person as are the various ingredients of your own healing recipe. My hope is that this book will help you accept the challenge of being in charge of your cancer recovery and to start your journey or help you continue on your present journey with more conviction and confidence.

The real turning point for my healing came after my first "metastatic scare" in March 1996, approximately six months after finishing chemotherapy. After a full evaluation, my doctors told me it was "nothing," but I fell apart during the medical work-up. At that time, I finally could clearly see that my usually submerged fears of what horrible thing was coming next in my life were preventing me from both simply enjoying today and also from reaching my fullest potential as a human being. I made the decision that I could fully accept the possibility that my body might die from cancer (we still all die from something), but I was no longer going to allow cancer to kill my spirit, too—in other words, I would not allow cancer to kill me twice! In an instant, all my anger over this latest cancer was gone, and my fears of what's coming next in life were gone, too.

In addition, I had spent a lifetime telling myself I was extraordinarily fortunate to have survived my childhood cancer, always moving forward in life by putting a positive spin on everything and both accepting and meeting challenges with determined optimism. Finally, at this point in my recovery, I allowed myself to both identify and grieve for all the losses I also had experienced by having cancer three times. I finally cried, and cried, and cried. When I was done crying, I realized that I had done a lot of forgiving and was ready for a new life. I was well on my way to being healed.

I am incredibly blessed to still have the gift of life, and also be considered cancer-free, after experiencing three separate cancer diagnoses. I now know that everything I accomplished in my life before this most recent cancer was "in spite of" my cancer history, and everything I accomplish from this point forward will be "because of" my cancer history. God must have had a plan for my life that included sharing my dietitian's knowledge and cancer experiences with other people, although it took me 47 years (almost a half a century!) to arrive at that point.

I can't foresee the future. Cancer is sneaky; it may still come back. I can accept that possibility. I sleep well at night knowing I'm no longer trying to outrun cancer. I'm simply trying to live each day well with a sense of happiness, meaning, and contentment. The reality is, cancer or no cancer, we all have only today, in fact only this moment, to be living our life to its fullest. If cancer does return, I will be disappointed but not defeated. I believe all the changes I have made in my lifestyle have helped extend my life, although I acknowledge that fact cannot be proven. However, all the changes I have made have indisputably increased the quality of my life, a worthy goal in its own right. Finally, I know I have healed from the trauma of my cancer diagnoses, perhaps the most important benefit of all.

By sharing myself with you, I hope I've given you both "information and inspiration" to make your cancer journey meaningful. I wish you all the best for a full recovery, optimal health, and most importantly, the healing of your spirit.

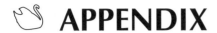 # APPENDIX

MY WEBSITE - www.CancerRD.com

When I first wrote and published my book, *A Dietitian's Cancer Story*, in 1997, my boys immediately both said, "Mom, now that you have a book, you need to be on the Web!" In 1997, I only had a vague idea of what they meant by that comment.

They helped me organize and develop the first content for my website. It very quickly evolved from simply being a means of selling my book to becoming a destination on the Internet for people looking for reliable and helpful information regarding nutrition and cancer. I keep adding new information every month, so come visit my Web site regularly. I post answers on my Web site to some of the many questions I receive. I am including some of the most frequently asked questions with my answers in this latest edition of my book. My answers can provide general information only and are not individualized medical or nutritional advice.

The most frequently asked question I receive is "What do you and your family really eat?" I have posted two weeks of menus, complete with all recipes, on my website. The recipes can be printed on various sized recipes cards or regularly sized paper. These are family-tested recipes that follow the nutritional guidelines I discuss in my book. I post new recipes every month, so check my website frequently for new ideas.

In addition, my website includes many links to other Internet resources containing reliable and beneficial information of importance to cancer patients and their support team. To date, people from 68 countries have visited my website, finding helpful and reliable information about nutrition and cancer, in addition to ordering information for *A Dietitian's Cancer Story* and its Spanish translation, *Historia De Cáncer De Una Dietista*.

I owe many thanks to my two sons for sharing their vision for my book. They gave me the idea (and the push) to reach my readers using this new technology in addition to the traditional printed book. Thanks, guys, I love you both!

In addition, I deeply thank my husband for patiently teaching me how to use the computer for word processing, which I did not know how to do before writing this book or the text for my Web site. He was always helpful about bailing me out when the computer gremlins would sneak in and cause such problems that I wanted to quit. Thanks, honey, for all that and much, much more. I love you, too!

Q—I have just been diagnosed with cancer. What steps do you suggest I take?

A—1) First have a good cry with a close friend or family member. There is even a book with this title; *First you Cry* by Betty Rollins, perhaps the first published personal account of surviving a disease that wasn't talked about years ago. Ms. Rollins is still alive, 20+ years after her first diagnosis, and the book has even recently been republished.

2) Then remember that someone somewhere has survived your type and stage of cancer. Read the book *50 Essential Things to do When the Doctor Says "It's Cancer!"* by Greg Anderson, who was told he has 30 days to live after a lung cancer diagnosis nearly 15 years ago!

3) Choose "active hope." Surviving this disease may be the "biggest project of your life, for your life." I cannot overemphasize this. Ask yourself and your medical team members "What can I do to help myself?" Even if you only change the odds two percent by being an equal partner in your care, you might be tipping the scale from 49 percent to 51 percent for long-term survival. Think of the psychological power that comes from being part of the majority!

4) Put together your whole support team and delegate what needs to be done (from taking the kids to after-school activities, meals, to finding a doctor). This is not the time to be shy. People really want to help you, but they may need to take direction from you. Read Amy Harwell's book *When Your Friend (or Relative) gets Cancer*. Another book by a cancer survivor who beat slim odds for survival that gives you hundreds of ideas how to have friends be helpful.

5) Get as many medical opinions as you need to make an informed decision about the choices you have for treatment—don't be shy about this! There are very few gold standards in cancer therapy. Make sure your additional opinions are from doctors who did their oncology training at different medical centers. Cancer survivor Steve Dunn has a good website to learn how to how to search the Internet for information about your cancer (www.cancerguide.org)

6) Choose a doctor(s) who is truly supportive of your goals and gives you hope. I cannot overemphasize this enough!

7) There is increasing scientific evidence that what you bring to the equation can help you survive longer and at the very least improve your quality of life. No one knows the complete answer to how to survive cancer, but activities such as participating in support groups, prayer, meditation, nutrition, exercise, and laughter (as a starting points) all may contribute their share to increasing your odds for long-

term survival. There is not a magic bullet (not any conventional therapy nor any dietary supplement) for full recovery from cancer. It requires a comprehensive or holistic approach to achieve full physical, emotional, mental, and spiritual recovery.

8) Request a consultation with the Registered Dietitian (RD) at your cancer center or clinic early after your diagnosis. Don't wait until you have lost or gained significant weight or developed side effects from your treatments that will impact your nutritional intake. Ideally, the RD should assess your nutritional needs in a proactive, in-depth, and individualized manner. She (he) will help you plan how to maintain the best nutritional status possible during active cancer treatments, manage (or even prevent) potential side effects from therapies, and then help you with information and motivation for choosing foods that may help increase your chances for long-term survival.

9) After you have chosen your treatment goals and path, believe in your choice with 1,000 percent conviction! I cannot overemphasize the power of belief. Do not worry that that your path is very different from the next person's. You both can achieve success. Recovery paths will be unique, just as you are unique. In addition to different conventional therapies (surgery, chemotherapy, or radiation), you may feel that certain teas and yoga are right for you, but the next person may choose T'ai Chi and meditation to supplement their conventional cancer therapy. There is more than one path to the mountain top!

10) When friends and relatives bring you information about various alternative treatments for cancer (and they will—I have grocery bags full of audiotapes and literature that people sent or brought me), first thank them for caring so deeply for you. Then tell them you will call them if you want more details about the particular product or treatment about which they brought you information. These choices are yours and yours alone to make—don't permit yourself to be pressured. Although there are many books on alternative therapies for cancer, my first choice of books is still Michael Lerner's *Choices in Healing*.

11) Read, read, read and be the patient with 10,000 questions (this is true for both conventional and alternative cancer therapies). Don't take any one source of information as the "gospel" truth, particularly

if that source has a financial interest in the product or procedure.

12) You will finally reach a point where you don't want or need any more information. That's OK! Then it's time to feel comfortable with the choices you have made for your recovery efforts and turn the outcome over to your faith. If I die from cancer, I will do so at peace knowing that I gave it my all; I looked under every stone and tried everything that made sense to me. In the meantime, I sleep well at night knowing that I am trying to help someone else have an easier cancer journey than I had.

Frequently Asked Question #2

Q—Do you ever "cheat" on your diet?

A—I count on someone asking me this question whenever I speak, and it does not matter if the audience is composed of cancer survivors or dietitians! This is a very common question and concern, particularly during the holiday season and stressful times such as after the terrorist events of September 11, 2001.

First of all, I will say that I believe wholeheartedly in my diet as a means of helping my body minimize the risk of cancer recurrence. I now look at everything I eat in a very mindful way, asking myself, "How does this food nourish me? How does it promote my recovery?" By asking myself these questions, I am acknowledging that food nourishes both the body and the soul.

After asking myself those two questions and deciding that a Christmas cookie is what I "need" to nourish my soul, I can then ask myself "How much do I need to eat to satisfy that need?" This technique may sound very tedious, and certainly not spontaneous, but it has permitted me to still enjoy the foods that are actually important to me and has also helped me maximize my intake of foods with anti-cancer potential. In other words, I "still have my cake and eat it, too," however, now I am satisfied with only one cookie instead of eating half the box in one sitting!

I invite you to try this method of eating during the next month. You may find that you have been eating most foods on "autopilot," without really thinking about how they can affect your recovery from cancer. Once you get in the habit of thinking of foods as important to nurturing your recovery, you will appreciate the title of a cookbook called *Life Tastes Better than Steak*, a vegetarian cookbook written for people with severe heart disease for whom medications and surgery have not worked or are not an option. Think about how you would title that book for yourself the next time you are faced with a food decision at a holiday party.

Frequently Asked Question #3

Q—What do you eat for snacks?

A—What do I snack on between meals? I am frequently asked this question during the Q & A period following my presentations. I do eat between meals two to three times each day.

Here are some of my favorite snacks:
- Dry roasted soy nuts (approximately two tablespoons) I do measure these because they are sooo good that it is easy to get carried away!
- A few almonds (five to six)
- A few Brazil nuts (one to two)—a good source of the anti-oxidant mineral selenium and a food plant source of omega-3 fatty acids
- Soynut butter (approximately one Tbsp.) on some whole grain crackers or an apple half
- Hummus (approximately two tablespoons) on some whole grain crackers or as a dip with some fresh veggies like red pepper strips, baby carrots, cauliflower or broccoli florets
- Fresh fruit—any kind
- Dried fruit—raisins, peaches, pears, figs, dates, apples, pineapples, cherries, cranberries, blueberries, prunes
- Vanilla yogurt on top of frozen raspberries, blackberries, or blueberries—top with approximately one Tbsp. of flaxmeal
- Air-popped popcorn—or the microwave variety that is the most reduced in fat content
- Pretzels—fat-free (I love the fat-free mustard pretzels by RoldGold.)
- Guiltless Gourmet™ baked chips with salsa or bean dip—I love these!
- Quaker Toasted Oatmeal® Squares—no milk—I eat them plain for a slightly sweet crunchy snack

And my favorite snack—because even I NEED some chocolate now and then—is frozen bing cherries, blackberries, or raspberries in a bowl drizzled (not drenched!) with Hershey's chocolate syrup. This is entirely fat-free and adds only a few calories from the chocolate syrup.

Frequently Asked Question #4

Q—What are your views about sugar for cancer patients? Does it "feed" tumors? Should I avoid it in any form?

A—I have a pretty simple approach to this controversial topic. Upon finishing my chemotherapy in 1995, I made the decision that I wanted everything going in my mouth to contain biochemical molecules that help with the cancer fighting process in my body. It is controversial whether sugar causes or promotes cancer, however I have

---

A Dietitian's Cancer Story

never seen one shred of data that indicates sugar prevents cancer.

So since sugar-laden foods (most processed dessert and bakery type items, candy, ice cream, many fruit juices to name a few examples) clearly take the place of calories from foods which have components with multiple anti-cancer activities, I do not want sugar-containing foods filling me up.

Whole fruits have many cancer-fighting phytochemicals, so I would not recommend limiting them. Many fruit juices on the market today are mostly apple or pear juice which have lower amounts of these important phytochemicals. When I drink juice, it is orange juice (great source of vitamin C and folic acid), pink grapefruit juice (good source of lycopene) or vegetable juices like carrot juice (abundant source of beta-carotene and other carotenoids, tomato juice (very good source of lycopene and vitamin C), or mixed vegetable juice (very good source of phytochemicals too numerous to name or count). Between meals, I also drink lots of unsweetened iced green tea and water.

After changing my diet to contain foods that I mention in my book, I completely lost my taste for "needing" desserts or other sweet items. I do occasionally have a cookie or something like that, but I never eat the whole box any more!

Hope this is helpful perspective. Best wishes to you for good health!

Frequently Asked Question #5

Q—The phytochemical shake you feature in your book makes three cups. Is that really just one serving? If so, can I drink some of it later? Does it keep in the refrigerator? Have you ever tried freezing it?

A—Yes, the entire recipe is one serving. I drink about half right away and then put the other half in an insulated coffee mug and sip the remainder through a straw over the next hour or so. It is all I have for breakfast and I drink this usually six days every week. (In contrast, my younger son drinks an even larger shake—about four cups—for breakfast in five minutes, plus a huge bowl of cereal, milk and fruit—I'm not kidding!)

Yes, it can be refrigerated, but it both thickens (due to the free water in the soymilk and juice being absorbed by the wheat bran and mucilage in the flax seeds) and separates. Many people have written to tell me they drink half of the shake in the morning and then the other half at a later time. They solved these issues by simply stirring in a little more juice when they were ready to drink it later, and then it is perfect!

Other people have written to say they make it up in bulk, and freeze it in one cup portion sizes for ease of handling when thawing. It needs to be thawed and then mixed with some additional liquid of some type to thin it down for the same reasons explained above. It can also be frozen in icecube trays and a single frozen cube enjoyed as a snack.

Frequently Asked Question #6

Q—My blender won't blend the carrots. Can you tell me what kind of blender you are using? Do you have other suggestions?

A—I have heard this from several people. I would suggest any one of the following changes:
• use baby food carrots,
• steam the raw carrots first,
• use thawed frozen carrots, or even
• use cooked sweet potatoes.

The carotenoid content (beta-carotene, alpha-carotene and many others) are stable in heat and food processing, with light cooking actually increasing the availability of the carotenoids for absorption during digestion.

I used the Oster Kitchen Center's blender attachment for three years with no problems at all. I now own a Vita-Mix. They are very expensive, but I have to admit to loving it! Magazines like *Consumer Reports* will have articles reviewing the capabilities of blenders. Information about the power of blenders can also be found on the Internet using any search engine.

Good luck and happy blending!

Frequently Asked Question #7

Q—Can herbs interact with any of the chemotherapy drugs?

A—Just one example of this potential problem is the very popular herb St. John's Wort, commonly consumed for mild depression. St. John's Wort can increase the type of enzymes in our body that have the function of metabolizing drugs, thus lowering levels of these drugs in our bloodstream. Several chemotherapy drugs are metabolized by these enzymes. Concurrently taking St. John's Wort can have the potential to lower the level of these chemotherapy drugs, thus possibly reducing their effectiveness.

Several examples would be Tamoxifen, Cytoxan, Etoposide, and Vincristine. *The Herb-Drug Interaction Handbook* by Sharon Herr, RD, is an exceptionally thorough, up-to date source of these herb-drug interactions. More information about this helpful book and ordering information is available on the website www.herbdrug.org/.

It is vital that you always inform all of your health care professionals of any herbs and other dietary supplements you are consuming, so that the potential for any adverse interactions can be evaluated.

Frequently Asked Question #8

Q—Which herbs might cause problems with blood clotting?

A—Many common herbs and other dietary supplements can increase bleeding risk by increasing the time it takes blood to clot. This is especially important if you have a low platelet count, are taking the anti-coagulant drugs (like warfarin/Coumadin or heparin), NSAIDS (like Advil, Motrin, Ibuprofen), aspirin, COX-2 inhibitors (like Vioxx, Celebrex), or having surgery (Please Note—this list is not all-inclusive).

It is critical that you tell your health care providers (physician, pharmacist, dietitian, nurse, anaesthiologist, dentist, among others) about all of your medications and all types of your dietary supplements. They should check for potential interactions in order to lower the risk of possibly fatal complications. You may need to be taught to watch for signs and symptoms of increased bleeding (bruising, petechia, purpura, frank bleeding) and have some blood tests monitored (international normalized ratio—INR, prothrombin time—PT).

The American Society of Anesthesiologists recommends the discontinuation of all herbs at least two weeks prior to any surgery.

Some of the more common herbs and dietary supplements that have data (some human case studies, some in vitro laboratory studies) to show anti-coagulant and anti-platelet potential are the following (this list is not all inclusive):

- Angelica root
- Anise
- Arnica
- Bilberry Leaf
- Black Cohosh
- Borage seed oil
- Bromelain
- Celery

- Chamomile
- Clove
- Feverfew
- Fish oil (omega-3 fatty acids)
- Garlic
- Ginger
- Ginkgo biloba
- Horse chestnut
- Horseradish
- IP-6
- Licorice root
- Onion
- Panax Ginseng
- Papain
- Parsley
- Red clover
- Sweet clover
- Tumeric
- Vitamin E
- Willow bark

A highly recommended book to purchase for your home library is *Herb-Drug Interactions* by Sharon Herr, RD. Purchasing information is found at www.herbdrug.org/. There are many herb-drug interactions to be avoided. This book will easily help you identify them.

Again, I cannot overemphasize the importance of telling your health care providers about all of the dietary supplements (herbs, vitamins, minerals, and other over the counter products) that you are taking. Don't wait for them to ask you. Let the right hand know what the left hand is doing. It could save your life!

Frequently Asked Question #9

Q—Does decaffeinated green tea still have the health-promoting phytochemical called Epigallo-catechin-gallate (EGCG)? Where can one buy organic green tea?

A—According to information and data on Salada's website (www.greentea.com), not all methods to remove caffeine are equal in this regard. They share data which demonstrates that the method using water and effervescence retains about 95 percent of the original content of various catechins in green tea, including EGCG, compared to the method using ethyl acetate which retains only aproximately 30 percent of the ECGC.

Recommendation—be a label reader, and call or write the company of a product that does not share its decaffeinating method on the label to inquire about the method used. Take that opportunity to be an advocate and ask that they choose a method that retains more of the healthful catechins.

There are several sources of organic green tea, some are decaffeinated and some are not. Ask at your local grocery or natural foods store or look on the Internet using any search engine and the terms organic green tea.

Frequently Asked Question #10

Q—I understand that eating fish, particularly fish high in omega-3 fatty acids like salmon, is healthy for our bodies. Yet I have heard that eating salmon may be harmful to our environment from the over-fishing of wild fish and also degrading effects from fish-farming plus I have concerns about not consuming mercury or other environmental contaminants. Can you clarify this confusion, and what type of salmon do you eat?

A—I have recently starting reading more information on this important topic. I do think it is important to consider both what is healthy for our body and also what is healthy for our planet when we make our food choices. As with everything, this question brings us to a complex area of study that is still being researched.

There are several very good resources for finding up-to-date information to help you make informed seafood purchasing decisions. I recommend looking at information on the following Web sites:

Monterey Bay Aquarium - www.montereybayaquarium.org

Environmental Defense Fund - www.oceansalive.org

Marine Stewardship Council - www.msc.org

Based on their recommendations, I now try to make sure I am buying Alaska salmon, which has very healthy wild populations. Most canned salmon is Alaskan salmon. Start asking questions at your fish store and in restaurants to show your concern about these important issues!

Q—I am currently taking Tamoxifen. My daughter heard on TV that I should be eating soy to make it work more efficiently. Do you know of any studies verifying this information?

A—Yes, I am familiar with two well-designed research studies that have shown increased benefit for lab animals with induced ER+ breast cancer when given both Tamoxifen and soy together. That means fewer breast tumors, smaller tumors, even regression of breast tumors in one study for the rats fed both Tamoxifen and a soy food called miso. I will give a short description of each of the studies below.

The first study by Gotoh et al., published in the *Japanese Journal of Cancer Research* 89(5):487 98, 1998, is a rat study in which all of the rats were given a chemical which induces ER+ breast cancer. The rats were then observed for their breast cancer (ER+) development (this is a prevention study) while receiving one of 4 different treatments in addition to their baseline diet:

(1) a control group which received no further treatments,
(2) a group which only received Tamoxifen,
(3) a group which only received miso (a soybean paste commonly eaten daily in Japan),
(4) a group which received both Tamoxifen and miso.

The rats given Tamoxifen and miso together had a response that showed dramatically fewer numbers of tumors per rat and also decreased size of tumors compared to all of the other treatment groups. The reduction observed was actually synergistic (*i.e.* 1+1=3), meaning that combining the miso and tamoxifen together produced an even larger response than by adding the percent reductions seen in the groups that received either tamoxifen and miso alone when comparing the results to the control rats which received no tamoxifen or miso.

Reported in this same research paper by Gotoh, a different experimental rat study observed rats that already had ER+ breast cancer. These rats were given Tamoxifen or Tamoxifen + miso together. These rats then were compared to rats given nothing by measuring the growth of their breast cancer tumors after a defined period of time. This experiment showed that the rats who received the combination of Tamoxifen plus miso were the only treatment group that actually had their breast tumors decrease in size instead of continuing to grow as did the tumors in the other two groups.

The second study entitled *Consumption of Soy Products May Enhance the Breast Cancer Preventive Effects of Tamoxifen* by Andreas I. Constantinou. et al,. at the University of Illinois, Chicago, IL was recently presented at The American Association for Cancer Research in March 2001.

Four groups of 20 female mice were treated with an agent (DMBA) that produces ER+ breast cancer plus the following test agents fed into their usual diet:

1) no treatment (DMBA control);
2) Tamoxifen
3) soy protein isolate (SPI)
4) Tamoxifen + SPI.
5) A fifth group of 10 female mice was fed the basal diet without being exposed to DMBA.

Tamoxifen was effective in reducing mammary tumors per mouse by 29 percent. A 37 percent reduction in tumors/mouse was evident in the group that was fed SPI, and a 62 percent reduction in the group that was fed Tamoxifen + SPI (this shows an additive effect—*i.e.* 1+1=2). The length of time it took for tumors to develop was significantly increased only in the Tamoxifen + SPI group. None of these treatments showed any effect in the rate of animal growth or caused any toxicity.

These two studies clearly showed increased benefit to the rats or mice given Tamoxifen plus a soy food (miso or isolated soy protein) over the rats given Tamoxifen or soy alone when compared to the control animals. Both studies showed clear preventive advantages to this combination and the Gotoh study showed benefit to rats in treatment for breast cancer as well.

Please note that extrapolating conclusions from animal experiments to humans is not perfect science. It is not known at this time if women with breast cancer who are taking Tamoxifen will have this same response when consuming soy with Tamoxifen, as "rat science" is not always translatable to humans. It is also not known if women taking Tamoxifen as a preventive agent should be consuming soy-foods to enhance that effect expected from Tamoxifen alone. A recommendation cannot be made until this combination is tested in humans. However, these results look promising. I consumed one to three soy foods per day the entire five years that I was on Tamoxifen after my 1995 breast cancer (October 1995 through October 2000) without a recurrence of my cancer during that time. I continue to consume this same amount of soy foods on a daily basis.

Please consult with your personal health care professionals before making any decisions about your choices of therapy and nutritional intake. I recommend that you ask your physician and the dietitian at your own cancer center for their recommendations. Feel free to share these references. Also ask for additional references to research that may be even more current than these as you gather information in order to make the best-informed decision possible in this world in which all research data are not yet available for cancer survivors.

Frequently Asked Question #12

Q—Should women with ER+ breast cancer consume flaxseeds and flax oil that contain the phytoestrogens called lignans?

A—There is a recent preliminary small human study showing that ingestion of 25 grams of ground flaxmeal per day in women with newly diagnosed post-menopausal ER+ breast cancer decreases biological markers of tumor growth the same amount as the anti-estrogen drug Tamoxifen during the time period between diagnosis and surgery. Tamoxifen treatment was not compared directly to flaxmeal in this study. The data are compared from two separate studies. In addition, this is such a small and early study that no recommendations for treatment with flaxmeal can be made based on these data. Much larger and longer head-to-head clinical trial studies in women would need to be done to offer this as a treatment option. However, these data look very promising that flaxmeal is not only safe but also potentially effective as a nutritional means for helping to treat ER+ breast cancer.

Please thoroughly discuss the pros and cons of ingesting flaxseeds as part of your dietary intake with your Oncologist and Registered Dietitian at your cancer center. Feel free to share the following reference for this data:

Biological Effects of Dietary Flaxseed in Patients with Breast Cancer. Abstract from the San Antonio Breast Cancer Symposium - December 2000, Thompson LU, Li T, Chen J, Goss PE Nutritional Sciences, University of Toronto, Toronto, ON, Canada; Medical Oncology, Princess Margaret Hospital, Toronto, ON, Canada.

I have seen no data yet showing the results of using flaxseed meal in conjunction with Tamoxifen. Dr. Thompson hopes to conduct experiments with this combination in the future.

I have been consuming one to two tablespoons of ground flaxseed meal daily since 1995 without a recurrence of my ER+, post-menopausal breast cancer.

Frequently Asked Question #13

Q—What can be done to relieve the fatigue I am still experiencing since my cancer therapy has been completed? Will any dietary supplements help me?

A—The reasons why cancer patients experience fatigue, even during the recovery phase, are multi-factorial and still being identified. I do not know if just adding any dietary supplements would do the trick all by itself.

I can say that for three years during the 10-year period between my two breast cancers I experienced overwhelming and debilitating fatigue. No physical reason could be found. I wasn't depressed. I just lived with it, and eventually the fatigue slowly lifted.

However, interestingly, although I experienced the same level of fatigue during both sessions of chemo (1984 and 1995), my recovery after the 1995 chemo was much more rapid and complete. I do not really know why that is so, nor do my doctors venture a guess. My best guess though is that my sustained level of high energy is due to my holistic approach to recovery this time—physical, mental, emotional, and spiritual. Yes, I do take a few supplements as I describe on pages 63 and 64, but I really doubt that my boundless energy is due to them alone.

If I had to pick a few changes that I think have made the most difference in energizing me (i.e., eliminating my fatigue), they would be the following, and in this order:
1) diet,
2) regular exercise,
3) connections and service—by that I mean my involvement with and commitment to helping others, in other words, serving others in need and not dwelling (too much) on my own problems,
4) stress reduction strategies like meditation, yoga, Qi gong, prayer, and
5) including lots of fun in my life, too.

Please be sure to discuss your fatigue with your oncologist so that any potentially treatable physical reasons for your fatigue may be identified and treated appropriately. In addition, please ask to speak to the registered dietitian at your cancer center. She will help you with many of these strategies that I have suggested and may also be able to advise you on the careful addition of appropriate supplements to your diet.

Two Web sites to visit for additional information on cancer fatigue include:
Oncology Nursing Society (www.cancerfatigue.org/)
BreastCancer.org (www.breastcancer.org)

A wonderful and helpful CD to combat cancer fatigue is available to purchase at www.healthjourneys.com.

Q—I have received conflicting advice regarding the use of supplemental antioxidants like vitamin C during my chemotherapy and radiation therapy. (1) Should I avoid them or take them? (2) Does this concern extend to the ingestion of foods containing high levels of antioxidants, like any food (such as an orange or orange juice) that has a high amount of vitamin C?

A—The use of various dietary supplements (vitamins, antioxidants, herbs, etc) by people with a cancer diagnosis is very common. Some reasons given for their use include:

1. Relieve unpleasant symptoms from the disease itself or side effects from the treatments,
2. Protect normal healthy cells from side effects produced by treatments,
3. Enhance healing after surgery,
4. Augment the effects from conventional cancer treatments,
5. Prevent recurrence of the original cancer and/or a new primary tumor,
6. Detoxify the body both during therapy and recovery.
7. Enhance the immune system

All of the above reasons have some intuitive merit. However, data from well-designed research studies are not plentiful to help guide choices of dietary supplements for a particular type and stage of cancer, dosing, timing, interactions with other therapy/drugs, etc. The number of products available in a health food store and for sale on the Internet is mind-boggling. Where to start? Where to stop?

I consider the concern regarding the use of antioxidants during cancer therapy the most controversial question in nutritional oncology at this time. Does the ingestion of dietary supplements that are antioxidants (such as vitamin C, vitamin E, selenium, and many others) increase, decrease, or have no effect on the potential benefits of chemotherapy, radiation therapy, and other biological or hormonal therapies?

These supplements are often recommended by popular books and some individual health care practitioners to use during cancer therapy in order to help protect the body's normal cells from the harmful side effects of chemotherapy and radiation. While this outcome is certainly desirable, the real question is how this practice might affect the potentially beneficial result intended from the use of chemotherapy or radiation therapy (i.e., help extend life with an acceptable level of quality of life). One mechanism of killing cancer cells is the generation of a massive amount of free radicals within the cancer cell by various chemotherapy drugs and radiation in order to disrupt replication and growth of the cancer cells. Thus there is concern by many oncologists that consuming additional supplemental antioxidants, which eliminate free radicals, may potentially reduce the effectiveness and defeat the very purpose of choosing to undergo conventional cancer therapies like radiation and chemotherapy.

Much research still needs to be done to evaluate this question in clinical trials (human data). Although preliminary research has been done in both in test tubes and animals, human testing is the only way to really know how the addition of various dietary supplements to a conventional cancer therapy will affect survival and quality of life.

In the meantime, the question of what to do still looms.

The best advice I can give you is to read, read, read (cross check everything—do not believe everything you read!), and be the patient with 10,000 questions. Determine your goals and then use the questions I have outlined in my "Decision Tree" (on page 61 to 62) as a springboard for being an informed and savvy cancer patient. Never use one source of information as your only source of information, particularly if that source has a financial interest in the product being sold! Invest much more research time deciding what to put into your body than you have in the past when buying a home or car. You are trying to choose a course of action that offers reasonable hope, instead of hype, or even possible harm.

Ultimately, the choice of what to do is a personal one. However, I strongly recommend discussing possible choices regarding the use of dietary supplements with members of your oncology team, particularly your physicians, dietitian and pharmacist. Ask them to share their thought process and references that have led to their recommendations. Also ask them to help you understand and interpret the scientific strength of advice, articles or information you may have found in various books, from the Internet, or from other practitioners.

Some books, articles, and web sites to read as starting points for information regarding the use of herbs, vitamins, and other dietary supplements in cancer:

- *Antioxidants against Cancer*, Ralph Moss, PhD, Equinox Press, 2000.

- *Beating Cancer with Nutrition* (revised), Patrick Quillan, PhD, 2001.

- *Choices in Healing—Integrating the Best of Conventional and Complementary Approaches to Cancer*, Michael Lerner, PhD, MIT Press, 1994.

- *Herbal Medicine, Healing & Cancer*, Donald Yance, Keats Publishing, 1999.

- *Herbs against Cancer*, Ralph Moss, PhD, Equinox Press, 1998.

- *Fight Cancer with Vitamins and Supplements: A Guide to Prevention and Treatment*, KN. Prasad, PhD, and K.C.Prasad, MD, Healing Arts Press, Rochester, VT, 2001.

- *Natural Compounds in Cancer Therapy*, John Boik, Oregon Medical Press, Princeton, MN, 2001.

- *Tyler's Herbs of Choice—The Therapeutic Use of Phytomedicinals*, James Robbers, PhD, and Varro Tyler, PhD, ScD, Haworth Press, 1999.

- *Tyler's Honest Herbal: a Sensible Guide to the Use of Herbs and Related Remedies*, Tyler and Steven Foster, Pharmaceutical Products Press, New York, 1998.

- American Botanical Council—www.herbalgram.org

- Consumer Lab—www.consumerlab.com

- Center for Alternative Medicine Research in Cancer—www.sph.uth.tmc.edu/utcam/

- National Center for Complementary and Alternative Medicine (NCCAM)—http://nccam.nih.gov/

- Office of Dietary Supplements (NIH)—http://odp.nih.gov.ods/

- Quackwatch (Dr. Stephen Barrett)—www.quackwatch.com

- Supplement Watch—www.supplementwatch.com

- "Possible interactions between dietary antioxidants and chemotherapy", Labriola D, and R Livingston, Oncology (Huntingt) 1999 July;13(7):1003-8, discussion 1008, 1011-12. Comments in Oncology (Huntingt) 1999 Dec;13(12):1624, 1627-28, 1631.

- "Antioxidants in Cancer Therapy; their actions and interactions with oncologic therapies", Lamson, D and M Brignall, Alternative Medicine Review 4(5):304-329, 1999.

- *Nutrition and Cancer: An International Journal*, published by Lawrence Erlbaum Associates, Inc., 10 Industrial Ave., Mahwah, NJ 07430-2262, 201-236-9500. Your cancer center's library may have this journal. In addition, many articles or abstracts from the journal are available on the Internet through Medscape (oncology.medscape.com) and through PubMed (www.ncbi.nlm.nih.gov/PubMed/—search by the journal title)

There are additional books and Web sites in the Resources section

---

of my book. Inclusion here is simply meant as a source of information to evaluate further, not an endorsement.

In answering your second question regarding concern about the consumption of foods high in antioxidants, I know of no large body of research that would lead me to conclude at this time that any food should be specifically avoided during cancer therapy because of its high content of antioxidants. It is the ingestion of individual antioxidants in the isolated form of a pill, often in doses significantly higher than obtained from usual amounts of food sources, that is of greater concern. The consumption has now changed, in essence, from a nutrient level to a pharmaceutical (drug) level.

Proceeds from the sale of my books are donated to the Diana Dyer Cancer Survivors' Nutrition and Cancer Research Endowment that I have established at the American Institute for Cancer Research (AICR) in Washington, DC. I direct this endowment to exclusively fund research projects that will focus on defining nutritional strategies after a cancer diagnosis, either during treatment or recovery, which will optimize the chances for long-term survival.

The first research project that my endowment has helped to fund through AICR will be evaluating the outcome (*i.e.* the effectiveness of chemotherapy on extending life) of adding an antioxidant to a specific chemotherapy regime in humans. Much more research of this type should be funded by our government's National Cancer Institute to help cancer patients and physicians optimize cancer therapy.

Information regarding additional donations to this endowment or grant applications may be obtained from the Director of Development at AICR by calling 1-800-843-8114.

Frequently Asked Question #15

Q—Is there any new information for breast cancer patients who have ER+ tumors regarding the safety of eating soy foods?

A—The potential health benefits along with the safety of eating soy foods has been the subject of research since the early-to-mid 1990's, when soy foods became the newest trend as a "health food". Because the soybean contains a molecule, an isoflavone called genistein that has a structural similarity to the hormone estrogen, concern has been raised regarding the safety of soy food consumption for women who have already had a diagnosis of estrogen-responsive (ER+) breast cancer and also those who are at high risk for developing breast cancer, the question being would consumption of a food containing genistein potentially increase the growth of an ER+ breast cancer?

The November 2001 issue of the *Journal of Nutrition* contains a lengthy article reviewing 288 research studies regarding this very concern. It is entitled Soy for Breast Cancer Survivors: A Critical Review of the Literature. (*Journal of Nutrition* 131:3095S-3108S, 2001).

Here is the final paragraph from the 2001 article:
"The honest response to each of these diametrically opposed claims (soy foods are ok to eat versus avoid all soy foods) is that no convincing data exist to support either claim. In fact, there are strongly conflicting data regarding both. As such, if women (with or without breast cancer) enjoy partaking soy products, then it seems quite reasonable for them to partake of them. As with most things, moderation of intake is probably wise. In this regard, Asian soy intake may serve as a general guide for Western women."

Three references are cited in this article to define what amount of soy comprises a typical Asian soy intake. Native Japanese adults typically consume what is roughly equivalent to 1 to 1.5 servings (US measures) of traditional soy foods per day (i.e., tofu, miso, tempeh, soy milk, edamame, see Page 28 for serving sizes of typical soy foods).

In 2006, The American Cancer Society published its own review of the scientific research available on this same question (Soy for Breast Cancer Survivors, *CA Cancer J Clin* 2006;56:323-353). Here is their concluding statement:
"For the breast cancer survivor, current evidence suggests neither specific benefits nor harmful effects when soy is provided in the moderate amounts observed in most traditional Asian diets (no more than three servings per day) as part of a healthy diet...It is prudent to avoid the high doses of soy and soy isoflavones that are provided by more concentrated sources such as soy powders and soy isoflavone supplements."

A research study (not just a review of other research as were the two previously mentioned articles) published in late 2009 (Xiao, et al, Soy Food Intake and Breast Cancer Survival. *JAMA*, 2009; 302 (22): 2437-2443) examined and compared the soy food intake with breast cancer recurrence and death rates in a large population of Chinese women who are breast cancer survivors living in Shanghai. The data, collected for approximately four years, showed a reduced recurrence and death risk in those women who consumed higher intakes of traditional soy foods such as tofu.

The reduction in recurrence risk "maxed out" at an intake of 11 grams of soy protein per day, which when translated into food, could consist of approximately 1-1/2 cups of soy milk, or 1/2 cup of firm tofu, or 2/3 cup of edamame as examples (or appropriate combinations of various soy foods—check the nutritional labeling for the soy foods you purchase).

Women in the group with the highest intake of soy protein had a 29 percent lower risk of death during the study period, and a 32 percent lower risk of breast cancer recurrence compared to the breast cancer survivors who consumed the lowest intake of soy protein.

"The inverse association was evident among women with either estrogen receptor-positive or -negative breast cancer and was present in both users and nonusers of tamoxifen. This study suggests that moderate soy food intake is safe and potentially beneficial for women with breast cancer," the researchers write.

An accompanying editorial (Ballard-Barbash and Neuhouser, Challenges in Design and Interpretation of Observational Research on Health Behaviors and Cancer Survival. *JAMA*, 2009; 302 (22): 2483-2484) does raise cautions about extrapolating these data to breast cancer survivors living in the US who will have many differences from Chinese women born, raised, and living in China. However, the authors do conclude it is likely that soy foods such as those traditionally consumed in Asian diet are safe for breast cancer survivors and may provide benefit for reducing risk of recurrence and death from breast cancer.

After my second breast cancer diagnosis in 1995, I began consuming traditional soy foods made from soybeans (i.e., tofu and soy milk) on a daily basis for the first time in my life. I knew that soy beans contained a large array of molecules that have anti-cancer activity through multiple different mechanisms, although the molecule that has received the most attention (i.e., controversy) is the "phyto-estrogen" called genistein. To make a long story short, as both a breast cancer survivor and Registered Dietitian, I have been regularly following the research and talking to scientists since 1995 about the potential benefits and safety concerns of consuming this estrogen-like molecule in food, always coming down on the side of consuming it in the foods and amounts typical of an Asian diet (1-3 servings/day).

Has my soy food consumption helped reduce my risk of recurrence (either locally or as distant metastases)? Frankly, it is impossible to truly know if that is the case. However, as my oncologist told me more than 10 years ago, it is very clear to him that, based on my experience, soy foods are safe, and he encouraged me to "keep doing what I am doing."

Thankfully, science keeps marching on with data being accumulated to help cancer survivors make lifestyle choices to increase their odds for living a long and healthy life. The data from the 2009 *JAMA* study seems to support my decision back in 1995 to begin incorporating soy foods into my daily overall healthy diet. Perhaps this is a case of science catching up with me since I was making personal decisions that needed to be made before all the science was in.

Bottom line: I continue to feel comfortable both recommending and consuming soy foods on a daily basis. I consume 1-3 servings per day (nearly everyday) of traditional soy foods such as tofu, unsweetened soy milk, tempeh, edamame, roasted soy nuts or soy nut butter, and miso. Where possible, I consume organic soy foods, and I try to always purchase soy foods made from organic soy beans grown in the USA.

Bonus Recipes

The following four recipes are the most popular on the recipe section of my website www.CancerRD.com. However, there are many additional family-approved delicious and healthy recipes on my website and my blogs: www.DianaDyer.com and www.365DaysofKale.com. I keep posting more recipes as I develop them, so please visit my website and blogs regularly. All of these recipes use foods containing a wide variety of phytochemicals known to prevent or interrupt the cancer process.

Tabouli

Tabouli is my all-time favorite food. When my husband and I first made it during the 1970s using a recipe from the book *Diet for a Small Planet*, we could not stop ourselves and ate the entire bowl, which was six servings!

Although tabouli can now be purchased in the deli section of most grocery stores, making it from scratch is easy and truly the best!

Ingredients:

- 1-1/2 cups dry bulgar (find dry bulgar in the health food section of your grocery store or at a natural foods store)
- 4 cups boiling water
- 1 cup cooked, drained beans—garbanzo, lentil, or small white beans (can cook from scratch or use canned, pre-cooked beans)
- 2 cups fresh parsley, minced (can use your blender or food processor for this, or a chef's knife also works great). In the summer, I use half parsley and half fresh mint. Don't worry about the amount—more is better here.
- 2 - 3 bunches green onions, sliced, both white and green parts
- 3 - 4 medium tomatoes, chopped (in the off-season, I spend the money on the vine-ripened tomatoes for the best flavor)
- 1/2 cup or more fresh lemon juice
- 1/4 cup extra-virgin olive oil
- 1 tsp. salt

Directions:

- Pour the boiling water over the dry bulgar in a medium to large bowl and let sit ~1-2 hours until water is absorbed. Drain very well using a colander. Bulgar will now be light and fluffy.
- Once bulgar is done, mix all the ingredients together. Chill for several hours or overnight.

Beautiful to look at and absolutely delicious to eat! Enjoy!

Fresh Tomato Soup

I have been using this delicious recipe for nearly 25 years, inspired by a recipe I first found in the cookbook *American Wholefoods Cuisine* by Nikki and David Goldbeck.

Ingredients:

- 2-3 Tbsp. extra virgin olive oil
- 1 medium onion, chopped
- 3-4 cloves garlic, chopped (chop ~10 minutes prior to sautéing)
- 1 medium carrot, chopped into small pieces
- 1 medium red bell pepper, chopped into small pieces
- 1 stalk celery with leaves, chopped into small pieces
- 4 cups chopped tomatoes (~1-1/2 pounds)—I put all the skins and the seeds in the soup)
- 1 Tbsp. whole wheat flour
- 3 cups water or vegetable broth
- 1 - 2 Tbsp. fresh basil (green or purple is OK)
- 1 teaspoon salt (I use less)
- 1 teaspoon tomato paste if using out of season tomatoes (both regular or dried tomato paste work well)

Directions:

- Heat 1 Tbsp. olive oil in big soup pot. Add onion, garlic, carrots, peppers, celery and then sauté for ~5 minutes until onion is transparent.
- Add tomatoes and simmer gently for 10 minutes, mashing occasionally with a wooden spoon until soft and pulpy. Sprinkle flour over tomatoes and stir smooth.
- Add water and seasonings, bring to a boil, and then turn heat down to simmer uncovered for 20 minutes if soup is to be pureed or 30 minutes if not (this cooking time is important for both flavor development and also to increase the amount of the cancer-protective phytonutrient called lycopene that is released from the tomatoes).
- To puree or not is a personal choice. I puree about half of the soup in my blender to thicken it up a bit. Reheat (do not boil again) before serving, adding the last tablespoon of olive oil right before serving.

There are endless variations you can do on this basic soup recipe. I often add a few left over greens (cut into small strips) like chard or kale to the soup, some left over brown rice can be added, or even some white beans. I have even added about one cup of white cannellini beans to the blender when pureeing half the soup in order to thicken the soup and also add a good protein source.

Serve with a large green salad and muffins for a complete and filling meal.

Banana-Walnut Flax Muffins

Modified from a recipe in *The Amazing Flax Cookbook* by Jane Reinhardt-Martin, RD

Ingredients:

- 1-1/2 cup flour (I use white whole wheat flour or whole wheat pastry flour)
- 3/4 cup ground flaxseed
- 1/2 cup white sugar
- 1 teaspoon baking soda
- 1 whole egg
- 1/4 cup canola oil
- 1 cup smashed bananas (3 medium or 2 large)
- 1 teaspoon vanilla extract
- 2 Tbsp. non-fat plain yogurt
- 1/2 cup chopped walnuts

Directions:

- In large bowl, mix together flour, flaxseed, sugar and baking soda.
- In separate bowl, mix egg, canola oil, bananas, vanilla, and yogurt.
- Mix wet into dry ingredients.
- Fold in walnuts.
- Use paper muffin cups or spray the muffin pans with non-stick spray. Bake large muffins 20-25 minutes at 350 degree oven. Bake mini-muffins ~15 minutes at 350 degree oven.

Makes 12 muffins or 30 mini-muffins.

These muffins freeze easily, so make up a double batch to have plenty on hand for breakfast, snacks, or to serve with home-made soup at a future meal when you have less time to cook.

Black Olive Tapenade

If using a food processor, be careful not to over-process—the tapenade should retain some texture from the olives and capers. Experiment with different varieties of olives.

Ingredients:

- 3/4 cup Kalamata olives, pitted (or use a combination of olive varieties)
- 1-1/2 Tbsp. capers, drained
- 1-2 garlic cloves, finely minced
- 1/8 cup minced fresh parsley leaves (or scant 1 Tbsp. dried)
- 2 - 3 grinds of black pepper
- 2 Tbsp. extra virgin olive oil

Directions:

- Combine all ingredients except oil in a food processor.
- Slowly add the oil and pulse, retaining some bits of olive and caper for texture.
- Taste to adjust the seasonings if necessary.

When stored tightly covered in the refrigerator, this will keep well for a week or two. This recipe can easily be doubled if you have a standard size food processor.

Makes about 1 cup. Serve on crackers or fresh baguette slices. I also serve it with fresh vegetables, spread it on sandwiches, and even put a dollop on baked potatoes. Enjoy eating a very healthy traditional food from the Mediterranean area. Making tapenade from scratch is a snap and costs a fraction of purchasing it already made from the grocery store.

✑ RESOURCES

The resources listed below are ones that I have personally used. There are many other sources of information, especially for other types of cancer. My recommendation is to read, read, read. I'm a firm believer in obtaining second opinions; I never accept one source of information as "gospel" (particularly if that source has a financial interest in the suggested therapy). Note: Updated editions are available for many of these books.

Cancer

Love, Susan, M., M.D., *Dr. Susan Love's Breast Book*, Perseus Publishing, Cambridge, MA, 3rd edition, 2000. The "Bible" of information needed by breast cancer patients to intelligently talk to their doctors and make informed decisions.

Murphy, G.P., M.D., L.B. Morris, and D. Lange, The American Cancer Society's book, *Informed Decisions: The Complete Book of Cancer Diagnosis, Treatment, and Recovery*, Viking Publishers, New York, 1997. An encyclopedia-type book on everything you want to know about cancer. Although the book is huge, you can pick and choose sections to read that are relevant for you.

Alternative Medicine

Chopra, Deepak, MD—any of his books. The one I chose to read first, *Quantum Healing*, was difficult to read as a starting point. I needed to read it twice, with six months and several other books under my belt between readings. Then the ideas in this book made more sense to me.

Collinge, William, M.P.H., Ph.D., *The American Holistic Health Association Complete Guide to Alternative Medicine*, Warner Books, New York, 1996—good overview, includes multiple references, and each chapter concludes with the strengths and limitations of the particular therapy being discussed and guidelines on choosing a practitioner for that therapy.

Eisenberg, DM, et al., "Unconventional Medicine in the United States—Prevalence, Costs, and Patterns of Use", *New England Journal of Medicine* 328 (4):246-252, 1993. The article that really gave a "wake-up call" to U.S. medical clinicians regarding the extent to which various aspects of alternative medicine were being used by their patients without informing their doctors.

Fugh-Berman, Adriane, M.D., *Alternative Medicine: What Works—A Comprehensive, Easy-to-Read Review of the Scientific Evidence, Pro and Con*, Odonian Press, Tucson, Arizona, 1996. A very good easy-to-read overview (not just of cancer) aimed at the layperson, medical professional, and researcher, includes multiple scientific references.

Kabat-Zinn, Jon, Ph.D., *Full Catastrophe Living*, Delacorte Press, New York, 1990. There are zillions of books on meditation. This is one that explains it well and gives many case examples of how the incorporation of mindful meditation into daily life has improved the health of average Americans. Helpful cassette tapes developed by the author are also available.

"The Magic of Healing—from Prevention to Renewal"—The Eight Step Guide to Physical, Mental and Spiritual Well-Being. Developed by Drs. Deepak Chopra and David Simon. This is the course I took where I learned to meditate along with other aspects of Ayruvedic medicine. Available by certified instructors around the country. Call 1-800-757-8897 for more information.

Micozzi, MS, M.D., Ph.D., *Fundamentals of Complementary and Alternative Medicine*, Churchill Livingstone, Inc., 1996—very good in-depth explanations of the various alternative healing traditions with many scientific references for further reading.

Moyers, Bill, *Healing and the Mind*, Doubleday Publishers, 1993—the video is also available as seen on PBS in 1993, audio tapes, and resource guide by calling 1-800-336-1917, or write P.O. Box 2284, S. Burlington, VT 05407. A wonderful, inspirational, and award-winning PBS series. If you haven't seen it, get the tapes from the library.

Murray, Michael, N.D., and Joseph Pizzorno, N.D., *Encyclopedia of Natural Medicine*, Prima Publishing, Rocklin, CA, 1997, revised second edition. An extensively referenced book of the principles and applications of natural medicine by two naturopathic physicians from Bastyr University, a naturopathic college in Seattle, WA, that has an American Dietetic Association approved Dietetics undergraduate degree and a Dietetic Internship.

Qi—The Journal of Traditional Eastern Health and Fitness, A quarterly journal to educate the public about the benefits of Asian traditions of healing. Recommended by my Qi gong instructor as a resource for finding qualified Tai Chi and Qi gong instructors in your locality. Available at some large book stores or phone 1-800-787-2600.

Weil, Andrew, MD, *Spontaneous Healing—How to Discover and Enhance Your Body's Natural Ability to Maintain and Heal Itself*, Alfred A. Knopf, 1995. An overview with case examples of alternative approaches to healing and maintaining optimal health. Easy to read.

A very good book to start exploring in this field. His plan requires a commitment to lifestyle changes, effort, and time (hence the title for his newest book, *Eight Weeks to Optimum Health*).

Alternative Cancer Treatments

Austin, S, N.D., and C Hitchcock, MSW, *Breast Cancer: What You Should Know (but may not be told) about Prevention, Diagnosis, and Treatment*, Prima Publishing, Rocklin, CA, 1994—a very interesting synthesis of both medical and alternative information as a naturopathic physician (SA) tries to help his wife (CH) choose her treatments after being diagnosed with breast cancer. For the most part, it is balanced and thoughtful book.

Boik, John, *Cancer and Natural Medicine—A Textbook of Basic Science and Clinical Research*, Oregon Medical Press, 1996. THE textbook I was looking for—gives a very good introduction to the steps of the carcinogenic process and very detailed information on the research that has shown how various nutrients and natural products may effect this process. Those without an extensive medical and/or nutritional background will need to frequently use a medical dictionary.

Boik, John, *Natural Compounds in Cancer Therapy*, Oregon Medical Press, 2001. In-depth information about the top three dozen natural compounds with cancer-fighting activity. Again, a very technical book.

Lerner, Michael, Ph.D., *Choices in Healing—Integrating the Best of Conventional and Complementary Approaches to Cancer*, MIT Press, 1994. The BEST resource I've currently found that fairly and thoroughly discusses many, but not all, unproven therapies for cancer. This entire book is on the Internet at the following website (www.commonweal.org/canproj.html). I highly recommend this book.

There are now numerous books available on the use of alternative and complementary therapies for cancer patients. Here are a few of the new ones available. As per my previous recommendations, read, read, read, getting second and third sources or opinions about any treatment you consider for yourself.

American Cancer Society, *American Cancer Society's Guide to Complementary and Alternative Cancer Methods*, ACS, 2000.

Cassileth, Barrie PhD, *The Alternative Medicine Handbook: The Complete Reference Guide to Alternative and Complementary Therapies*, WW Norton & Co., 1999.

Gordon, James, MD and Sharon Curtin, *Comprehensive Cancer Care: Integrating Alternative, Complementary, and Conventional Therapies*. Perseus Books, 2001 (paperback edition).

Herbs

Craig, Winston, Ph.D., RD, *The Use and Safety of Common Herbs and Herbal Teas*, Golden Harvest Books, Berrian Springs, MI, 1996. A good overview.

Duke, James, Ph.D., *The Green Pharmacy*, Rodale Press, 1997. Fun to read. This book unfortunately has no references, but Dr. Duke is a highly respected botanist by both the academic and herbal communities.

German Government's *Commission E Monographs* on herbs and their efficacy and safety, etc., have recently been translated into English by The American Botanical Council. This information is considered the world's largest compilation of data supporting the safe and appropriate indications for using medicinal plants (order by calling 1-800-373-7105).

Herbalgram—The peer-reviewed journal of the American Botanical Council and the Herb Research Foundation—two very responsible organizations promoting accurate scientific research and education of the public about medicinal benefits and potential of herbs. Can be found at large bookstores, natural food stores and even some grocery stores. Published quarterly.

Keville, Kathi, *Herbs for Health and Healing*, St. Martin's Press, 1996—good section on cautions and considerations.

The Review of Natural Products (formerly *The Lawrence Review of Natural Products*)—an extensive series of unbiased, peer-reviewed, and referenced reviews of natural products that includes information on botany, history, chemistry, pharmacology, toxicology, summary, and references. Published by Facts and Comparisons, Wolters Kluwer Company, 111 West Port Plaza, Suite 300, St. Louis, MO, 63146-3098.

Taylor, Nadine, MS, RD, *Green Tea: The Natural Secret for a Healthier Life*, Kensington Books, 1998. A well researched book.

Tyler, Varro, Ph.D., Sc.D. and J Robbers, PhD, *Tyler's Herbs of Choice—The Therapeutic Use of Phytomedicinals*, Haworth Press, 1999 —a very thorough explanation of the clinical research on medicinal effects of herbs. The late Dr. Tyler was considered "the" leading scientific expert in this country promoting the safe and appropriate medicinal use of herbs. Organized by therapeutic indication—disease and/or organ function.

Tyler, Varro, Ph.D., Sc.D. and Steven Foster, *Tyler's Honest Herbal: a Sensible Guide to the Use of Herbs and Related Remedies*, Pharmaceutical Products Press, New York, 1998. Organized by herb.

Anderson, Greg, *50 Essential Things to do When the Doctor Says It's Cancer*, Plume Publishers, 1993. The best book to buy a friend early after their diagnosis. Each chapter is very short and succinct—easy to read when you're in a state of shock and/or simply frazzled.

Canfield, J, MV Hansen, P Aubery, and N Mitchell, RN, *Chicken Soup for the Surviving Soul*, Health Communications, Inc., Deerfield Beach, FL, 1996. A wonderful, hopeful, inspirational book. Buy it for a friend or relative with cancer.

Halvorsen-Boyd, Ph.D., Glenna and Lisa Hunter, Ph.D., *Dancing in Limbo—Making Sense of Life after Cancer*, Jossey-Bass Publishers, San Francisco, 1995. A very good description of the various stages of recovery, based on the personal experiences of both authors.

Harwell, Amy, *When Your Friend Gets Cancer—How You Can Help*, Harold Shaw Publishers, Wheaton, Illinois, 1987. The best book to buy yourself when you have a friend with cancer.

National Coalition for Cancer Survivorship, Hoffman, Barbara, Editor, *A Cancer Survivor's Almanac—Charting Your Journey*, Chronimed Publishing, 1996—the best guide for seasoned survivors —would be overwhelming on the day of diagnosis.

Siegel, Bernie S., MD, *Love, Medicine, and Miracles*—Dr. Siegel's first book. Many cancer patients say this book was a lifesaver. However, it is intense, and not every patient is ready early after his or her diagnosis to delve into Dr. Siegel's questions. Additionally, this book has been highly criticized by some cancer patients who believe Dr. Siegel is indirectly stating cancer patients' own negative thoughts and emotions may be "causing" their own cancers, although I didn't read it that way.

Siegel, Bernie S., M.D., *Peace, Love, and Healing—Bodymind Communication and the Path to Self-Healing: An Exploration*, Harper and Row, New York, 1989. Dr. Siegel's second book, an extension of his first.

Sternberg, Susan Wolf, *A Year of Miracles—A Healing Journey from Cancer to Wholeness*, Star Mountain Press, Ann Arbor, MI, 1996. This is an incredibly inspirational book written by a cancer survivor diagnosed with widely metastatic kidney cancer who sought out and combined the best that conventional and complementary medicine could offer her. She is alive and thriving eight+ years after her diagnosis!

The American Dietetic Association can offer assistance in the following ways:

Dietitian Referral Phone Line—1-800-366-1655

Dietitian Referral Internet Site—http://www.eatright.org

American Institute of Cancer Research Newsletter, AICR, 1759 R Street NW, Washington, D.C., 20009—information, recipes, and newsletter focusing on cancer and nutrition, including a new booklet called *Nutrition and the Cancer Survivor*. This non-profit research and education organization has been a pioneer in the area of nutrition and cancer. Get on their mailing list by calling 1-800-843-8114. Registered dietitians are available to answer general questions.

Brown, J. et al, "Nutrition During and After Cancer Treatment: A Guide for Informed Choices by Cancer Survivors," *CA, A Cancer Journal for Clinicians* 51(3):153-181, 2001

Eating Hints for Cancer Patients, National Institutes of Health, National Cancer Institute—recently revised. Ask your cancer center for a free copy or call 1-800-4-CANCER.

Keane, M, MS, and D. Chase, MS, *The What to Eat if You Have Cancer Cookbook*, Contemporary Books, 1997. A very good chapter on shakes and smoothies.

Mathai, Kimberly, MS, RD, *The Cancer Lifeline Cookbook*, Sasquatch Books, Seattle, WA, 2004. Highly recommended.

Nixon, Daniel, MD, *The Cancer Recovery Eating Plan—The Right Foods to Help Fuel Your Recovery*, Times Books, 1996. Overall, this is an informative and hopeful book with wonderful, healthful recipes.

Sattilaro, A. J., M.D., *Recalled by Life*, Avon Books, New York, NY, 1982. A physician's own story of his cancer diagnosis and subsequent change to a macrobiotic diet that he is convinced substantially extended his life. (He did subsequently die of recurrent prostate cancer.) I did not choose to go the full macrobiotic route, but this is the book that actually got me thinking seriously about making changes in my diet.

Weihofen, Donna, MS, RD, and C. Marino, MD, *The Cancer Survival Cookbook*, Chronimed Publishing, 1998. A wide selection of helpful recipes and information from an oncology dietitian at The University of Wisconsin Comprehensive Cancer Center.

World Cancer Research Fund and The American Institute for Cancer Research, *Food, Nutrition and the Prevention of Cancer: a Global Perspective*, AICR, 1997. Extensive information.

Newsletters which I Read

I am overwhelmed by the number of health and wellness newsletters available. Here are a few that I read regularly:

American Institute of Cancer Research Newsletter, AICR, 1759 R Street NW, Washington, D.C., 20009—free information and newsletter focusing on cancer and nutrition. Get on their mailing list by calling 1-800-843-8114. (Free but donations appreciated!)

Dr. Andrew Weil's Self Healing Newsletter—1-800-523-3296

Environmental Nutrition Newsletter—1-800-829-5384

Nutrition Action Health Letter, Center for Science in the Public Interest, Suite 300, 1875 Connecticut Ave., N.W., Washington, DC 20009-5728

Tuft's University Health & Nutrition Letter—1-800-274-7581

Vegetarian Nutrition and Health Letter, Loma Linda University, 1705 Nichol Hall, School of Public Health, Loma Linda, CA 92350

Vegetarian Journal, Vegetarian Resource Group, PO Box 1463, Baltimore, MD 21203

All of these newsletters and others like them (Harvard, Mayo Clinic, UC-Berkeley, Johns Hopkins, etc.) have a fee. Your local public library, medical system's patient education library, or even your own cancer center patient library may already subscribe to some of these so you could skim through them to look for articles of interest to you for free. In addition, there are certainly many additional informative newsletters for individual cancer types.

Internet Resources

It takes careful searching and lots of knowledge to interpret everything that is on the Internet. There are more hits on the Internet under the category "Alternative Medicine" than any other category, including many product marketing sites. In my opinion, these are some reliable places to start (all Web sites with http://):

Alternative Medicine Sources	www.pitt.edu/~cbw/altm.html
American Cancer Society	www.cancer.org
American Botanical Council	www.herbalgram.org
American Institute for Cancer Research	www.aicr.org
BreastCancer.Net	www.breastcancer.net
CancerGuide	www.cancerguide.org
Center for Science in the Public Interest	www.cspinet.org
ConsumerLab.com	www.consumerlab.com
Herb Research Foundation	www.herbs.org
MEDLINE (free access)	www.ncbi.nlm.nih.gov/entrez/query
National Cancer Institute	www.cancer.gov
NIH—Center of Alternative Medicine	nccam.nih.gov/
Office of Dietary Supplements	ods.od.nih.gov/databases/ibids.html
OncoLink (U of Penn)	www.oncolink.upenn.edu
Rosenthal Center for CAM	www.rosenthal.hs.columbia.edu/

Moss, Ralph, Ph.D., *Alternative Medicine Online*, Equinox Press, 1997. A book to help you get started looking at sites for alternative medicine on the Internet. I think about everything on the Internet very critically. Be cautious. Think about who is funding the web site and the potential for bias in the presentation of information.

Miscellaneous

National Cancer Institute—1-800-4-CANCER—call for free information about cancer, educational materials, and clinical trials available for your type and stage of cancer.

National Coalition for Cancer Survivorship—1-877-TOOLS-4-U—call for a free Cancer Survival Toolbox ™ containing three audio cassette tapes and workbook to help teach you self-advocacy skills as you prepare to participate in the fight for your life.

Dozens of medical journals devoted to various aspects of complementary and alternative medicine, intended for MDs and other health care professionals, have begun publication over the past several years. Check to see which ones are in the medical library of your doctor's hospital or cancer center. I purchase the following peer-reviewed journal frequently at my local large bookstore: *Alternative Therapies in Health and Medicine*, ed. Lawrence Dossey, MD.

"Living Dialogues" and "New Dimensions" shows on National Public Radio explore many aspects of complementary therapies to enhance health and wellness. Call your local public radio station to see if and what time these shows are aired in your locality.

Center for Alternative and Complementary Medicine (NIH)—1-888-644-6226

Food and Drug Administration (FDA) "MedWatch"—to report adverse reactions to drugs or dietary supplements, including herbs—1-800-332-1088 (you may call to "self-report").

The Herb Research Foundation operates a "Natural Healthcare Hotline" from which you may obtain information about herbs for a reasonable fee. Call 1-800-307-6267

Safetyalert.com—a Web site where you can find recall information about food and dietary supplements.

The following books are available with a study guide for CEUs for health care professionals from Helm Seminars and Publishing. To order, visit www.helmnutrition.com

• Collinge, William, M.P.H., Ph.D., *The American Holistic Health Association Complete Guide to Alternative Medicine*, Warner Books, New York, 1996

• Tyler, Varro, Ph.D., Sc.D., *Herbs of Choice—The Therapeutic Use of Phytomedicinals*, Haworth Press, 1999

• Tyler, Varro, *The Honest Herbal: a Sensible Guide to the Use of Herbs and Related Remedies*, Pharmaceutical Products Press, New York, 3rd edition, 1998.

Additional Helpful Books/Tapes

Bender, Sue, *Plain and Simple: A Woman's Journey to the Amish*, Harper Collins Publisher, New York, 1989. The book that profoundly influenced me to listen to my heart and inner voice while I was making the difficult decision to leave my previous professional position in the ICU.

Benson, Herbert, MD, *Timeless Healing: The Power and Biology of Belief*, Simon and Schuster, New York, 1997. The author of *The Relaxation Response* and founder of Harvard Medical School's Mind/Body Institute summarizes all the current data and knowledge that shows the importance, value, and benefits of our beliefs for promoting healing. Easy and powerful reading.

Breast Cancer: Surviving and Winning, a PBS documentary. Call your local PBS TV station asking when this will air (or re-air). A copy of the hopeful video can be purchased from the following website: www.survivingandwinning.com. (Twelve scientists and survivors, including me, are featured.)

Dossey, Larry, MD, Healing Words: the Power of Prayer and the Practice of Medicine, Harper Collins Publisher, 1993. I met Dr. Dossey and heard him speak in early April 1998. I hung onto his every word during his presentations and feel totally comfortable recommending his books.

Dyer, Wayne, Ph.D., Manifest Your Destiny: The Nine Spiritual Principles for Getting Everything You Want, HarperCollins, New York, 1997. So far I have only listened to the tapes of this book. They were truly inspirational and left me tingling with goosebumps. These tapes (or the book) deserve to be a part of every cancer survivor's healing journey when she/he is ready to tackle the "what to do with the rest of my life" question.

Halverstadt, A. and A. Leonard, Essential Exercises for Breast Cancer Survivors, Harvard Common Press, Cambridge, MA, 2000—a book devoted to guiding breast cancer patients back to full recovery through various exercises. Well researched with plenty of photos.

Naparstek, Belleruth—guided imagery cassette tapes entitled For People with Cancer and For People Undergoing Chemotherapy, Image Paths, Inc., 1-800-800-8661. I have had the opportunity to meet Belleruth Naparstek and participate as she guided the audience through an imagery session at a conference. Even though I was three years past my last diagnosis at the time, and thought I was finished with my healing, her imagery session was a profound experience and brought me even more healing. I highly recommend her tapes.

Nelson, M., Strong Women, Strong Bones, Putnam Publishing Group, 2000. The book that is quickly becoming the "Bible" for women to prevent and improve their osteoporosis. I wish I had this book and advice about how to improve my osteoporosis, which started with my premature menopause at age 34 from chemotherapy for my first breast cancer.

Siegel, Bernie, MD—many guided imagery and affirmation tapes available through his organization called ECaP. I have used several since 1995 and never fail to feel as though Bernie is actually holding my hand and telling me I can and will heal. These tapes have been very helpful. Dr. Siegel has a new web site at www.ecap-online.org, or call 1-814-337-8192 for more information.

High Fit—Low Fat Vegetarian, E.R. Burt, I.A.C.P., K.B. Goldberg, M.S., R.D., K.S. Rhodes, Ph.D., R.D., University of Michigan Medical Center, Ann Arbor, MI, 1996. Wonderful recipes.

Jane Brody's Good Food Book, W.W. Norton and Co., 1985.

Jane Brody's Good Food Gourmet, Bantam Publishers, 1990.

Jane Brody's Good Seafood Book, Balantine Publishers, 1994.

All of Jane Brody's cookbooks emphasize low fat eating, the significant reduction of the amount of meats eaten while increasing consumption of beans, whole grains, fruits, and vegetables. These are terrific cookbooks to start with if you're not ready to be 100 percent vegetarian yet.

Lickety-Split Meals for Health Conscious People on the Go!, Zonya Foco, RD, 1-888-884-LEAN. Great recipes, all of which have tips for making them meatless. I love the clever design of this book. It stands up on my kitchen counter with the recipe easy to read.

Life Tastes Better than Steak Cookbook, Gerry Krag, M.A., R.D. and Marie Zimolzak, D.T.R, Avery Color Studios, Marquette, MI, 1996. Great vegetarian recipes and what a profound title!

Magic Beans, Patti Bazel Geil, MS, RD, CDE, John Wiley and Sons, 1996. Terrific bean recipes. You are sure to find some that you and your family will love in this book.

Meatless Meals for Working People: Quick and Easy Vegetarian Recipes, D. Wasserman and C. Stahler, The Vegetarian Resource Group, P.O. Box 1463, Baltimore, MD, 1996.

Prevention magazine—I look forward to great new recipes each month.

Simple, Lowfat and Vegetarian: Unbelievably Easy Ways to Reduce the Fat in Your Meals!, Suzanne Havala, M.S. R.D., Vegetarian Resource Group, P.O. Box 1463, Baltimore, MD, 1994. This is more than just recipes—this is a book about how to eat this way in real life (from restaurants to amusement parks!).

The Simple Soybean and Your Health, M. Messina, Ph.D., V. Messina, R.D., and K. Setchell, Ph.D., Avery Publishing Group, Garden City Park, NY, 1994. A great overview of the potential health benefits of including soybeans in a diet with several good recipes for getting started.

Simply Soy: A Variety of Choices, K. Rhodes, Ph.D., R.D. and C. Sullivan, M.A. R.D., The Michigan Soybean Promotion Committee. This helpful booklet is out of print but is still available on the Internet. (search using the title)

Vegetarian Cooking for Healthy Living, M. Ter Meer, BS, and J. Galeana, MS, RD. Great recipes, easy to follow with common ingredients. 1-800-322-5679.

The Vegetarian Way: Total Health for You and Your Family, M. Messina, Ph.D. and V. Messina, MPH, RD, Crown Trade Paperbacks, New York, 1996. Very good information about vegetarian diets along with recipes.

Restaurant and Traveling Dining

Bartas, Jeanne. "Vegan Menu Items at Fast Food and Family-Style Restaurants, Part I." *Vegetarian Journal* Nov/Dec 1997. http://www.vrg.org/journal/vj97nov/97bvegan.htm

Bartas, Jeanne. "Vegan Menu Items at Fast Food and Family-Style Restaurants, Part II." *Vegetarian Journal* Jan/Feb 1998. http://www.vrg.org/journal/vj98jan/981fast2.htm

Bartas, Jeanne. *Vegetarian Menu Items at Restaurant and Quick Service Chains*. Baltimore: The Vegetarian Resource Group, 1997. A condensed version is available on the VRG web site: http://www.vrg.org/nutshell/fast.htm Order info: Send $4.00 to The Vegetarian Resource Group (see address below) and request the "Guide to Fast Food."

Duyff, Roberta Larson, MS, RD, CFCS. *ADA's Complete Food & Nutrition Guide*. Chronimed Publishing: U.S., 1996, Chapter 15: "Your Food Away From Home" and pp. 567-9 ("Eating Out The Vegetarian Way").

Kurleto, Betsey, RD, MA & Price, Beverly, RD, MA. *Nutrition Secrets for Optimal Health*. Farmington Hills, Michigan: Tall Tree Publishing Company, 1996, pp. 172-175 ("Dining Out").

Havala, Suzanne, MS, RD. *Simple, Lowfat & Vegetarian*. Baltimore: The Vegetarian Resource Group, 1994.

Havala, Suzanne, MS, RD. *Good Foods, Bad Foods: What's Left to Eat?* Minneapolis: Chronimed Publishing, 1998. Chapter 10: "Eating Out" and Chapter 12: "Traveling Light."

Levy, Linda & Grabowski, Francine, MS, RD. *Low-Fat Living for Real People*. New York: Lake Isle Press, Inc., 1994, pp. 77-92 ("Strategies for Eating Out").

Messina, Virginia, MPH, RD & Messina, Mark, PhD. *The Vegetarian Way*. New York: Crown Trade Paperbacks, 1996, pp. 263-70 ("The Vegetarian Traveler").

Pensiero, Laura, RD, Oliveria, Susan, ScD, MPH, with Osborne, Michael, MD. *The Strang Cookbook for Cancer Prevention*, pp. 338-45. New York: Penguin Putnam, 1998.

Warshaw, Hope S., MMSc, RD, CDE. *The Restaurant Companion: A Guide to Healthier Eating Out*. Chicago: Surrey Books, Inc., 1995.

Wasserman, Debra & Stahler, Charles. *Meatless Meals for Working People*. Baltimore: The Vegetarian Resource Group, 1996, pp. 11-22 ("Eating Out").

American Institute for Cancer Research (AICR)—For pamphlets, call 1-800-843-8114. *Cooking Solo* ("Meals on the Run" section), *Healthy Eating Away from Home*

Dixie USA, Inc. Call 1-800-233-3668 to order Nutlettes Plus® cereal or other vegetarian products

Musk, Maye, MS, MS, RD, web page: www.mayemusk.com or e-mail nutrition@mayemusk.com to request information on "nutritious food choices in restaurants."

The Vegetarian Resource Group—phone: (410) 366-VEGE *Vegetarian Journal's Guide to Natural Foods Restaurants in the US and Canada*. (To order, go to http://www.vrg.org/catalog/guide.htm or call above number.)

Vegetarian Times magazine (often has information on finding vegetarian food abroad). Look for at your local bookstore or library.

Note: Telephone numbers and Web sites change frequently. If you find that they are not correct when you read this book, please use telephone information or an Internet search engine to find the current contact information.

ORDERING INFORMATION FOR ADDITIONAL BOOKS

Additional copies of *A Dietitian's Cancer Story* may be obtained by several different means.

🍎 The book may be special ordered from any bookstore or by any library using the ISBN number: 978-0-9667238-3-0.

🍎 It is available for sale on many Internet book store sites, including Amazon.com. Search by my name or title.

🍎 I prefer that my book be ordered directly from the American Institute for Cancer Research (AICR). Ordering from AICR increases the amount of proceeds I can donate to AICR-funded research projects. Please call 1-800-843-8114 for current pricing and to order by credit card.

Bulk orders (10+) are priced lower. Please call AICR for further information.

Please visit my Web site and blogs frequently. I post great tasting, healthy recipes, my answers to many frequently asked questions, plus additional helpful research articles and Web sites for cancer survivors.

Diana Dyer, MS, RD
c/o Swan Press
PO Box 130221
Ann Arbor, MI 48113

Phone: 734-996-9260
Fax: 734-996-9260

Web Site: www.CancerRD.com

Blogs: www.dianadyer.com, www.365DaysofKale.com,
www.cancervictorygardens.com

🦢 About the Author

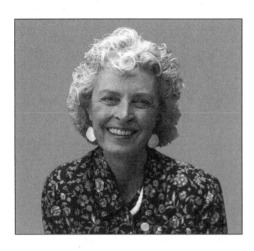

Diana Grant Dyer grew up in Toledo, Ohio. Her neuroblastoma was treated at The Toledo Hospital, Toledo, OH, and her two breast cancers were treated at Evanston Hospital, Evanston, IL, and The University of Michigan Comprehensive Cancer Center, Ann Arbor, MI.

She received her B.S. degree in Biology from Purdue University. Her M.S. degree in Nutritional Sciences and Dietetic Internship were completed at The University of Wisconsin and The University of Wisconsin Hospitals, respectively. In-between cancer diagnoses, she spent her entire career as a clinical dietitian working at several hospitals in the Midwest, specializing in nutritional care for the critically ill patient.

Diana has received the following awards:

Michigan Individual Public Relations Award
The Michigan Dietetic Association

Michigan Dietitian of the Year Award
The Michigan Dietetic Association

Distinguished Practice Award
*The Oncology Nutrition Dietetic Practice Group
of The American Dietetic Association*

Diana lives with her husband in Ann Arbor, Michigan. They have recently purchased property to start a small organic farm. Their two grown sons love coming home to help out and see what's new on the farm.